Aloe Vera

NATURAL WONDER CURE

JULIA LAWLESS AND JUDITH ALLAN

Thorsons

While the authors of this work have made every effort to ensure that the information contained in this book is as accurate and up to date as possible at the time of publication, medical and pharmaceutical knowledge is constantly changing and the application of it to particular circumstances depends on many factors. Therefore it is recommended that readers always consult a qualified medical specialist for individual advice. This book should not be used as an alternative to seeking specialist medical advice, which should be sought before any action is taken. The authors and publishers cannot be held responsible for any errors and omissions that may be found in the text, or any actions that may be taken by a reader as a result of any reliance on the information contained in the text, which is taken entirely at the reader's own risk.

Thorsons
An Imprint of HarperCollins*Publishers*
77–85 Fulham Palace Road,
Hammersmith, London W6 8JB
The Thorsons website address is: www.thorsons.com

Published by Thorsons 2000

10 9 8 7 6 5 4 3 2 1

A catalogue record for this book
is available from the British Library

ISBN 0 7225 3824 3

Printed in Great Britain by
Woolnough Bookbinding Ltd, Irthlingborough, Northants

To DR HAMISH ALLAN MBE

for his infinite kindness to all living beings

Contents

ALOE VERA

Acknowledgements

ALOE VERA

This book could not have been written without the following people: above all Celia and Brian Wright for their loan of scientific papers; and Nicholas Orosz for generous access to his library. Others who were of significant help were Dr Tom Reynolds of Jodrell Laboratories, Kew Gardens; Karen Masterson; Dr David Smallbone; Dr Vladimir Maikov; Natasha Hull for translating Russian texts; Mr Mistry; Maryk Vogel; John Knowlton; Joan Allan for her help with South African tribal lore; James Allan; Jane Moseley; Natasha Lawless; George Hull; Julia Hull; Ruth Dwornik; Dr Richard Dixey; Dr Amala Raman; Princess Helena Moutafian; Stephen Turoff; Mark and Natalie Foster; Robert Beer; Ruth West; Alan Hodgson; Yvonne Rawsthorne; Hetty Maclise; Murray Douglas; Gill Gannon; Catriona Mundle; Jenny Walden; Dorothee von Greiff; the Beresford family; Mandy Hon at Jukes Productions; Andy and Sally Stapley; Cara Denman; Dr Myrto Angeloglou; Anthony Dweck; Miss Carol Andrews; Assistant Keeper of the Department of Egyptian Antiquities at the British Museum; Marianne Winder and the staff at The Wellcome Institute; our editors at Thorsons, Jo Kyle, Victoria McCulloch, Barbara Vesey and Wanda Whiteley for their help and encouragement; and last but not least Rusky, the Pharaoh hound, for her patience.

Preface

I have always had a great love of plants, especially aromatic herbs and those species which have medicinal qualities. Aloe *vera* is not only an easy and extremely decorative plant to grow at home, it is also one of the most versatile and potent natural remedies available.

Aloe *vera*'s freshly cut leaves have enormous value as a home treatment for a wide range of common complaints, and this adaptability is reflected in the ever-expanding range of Aloe *vera* products which can be found on the market today.

I myself have experienced the dramatic healing potential of aloe in relation to skin care. Having suffered from an allergic skin rash for several months and trying a number of different natural treatments without success, the condition cleared up in less than a week after daily application with Aloe *vera* gel! I have come across numerous personal accounts of a similar and even more startling nature, where Aloe *vera* was able to bring about a seemingly miraculous recovery when all other medicines had failed. It is no wonder that one of the folk names for this remarkable plant is 'Miracle Worker'!

In writing this book I have been extremely fortunate to have been working with Judith Allan as co-author. Having grown up in southern Africa, one of her earliest recollections was of her grandfather's sub-tropical garden. He was a collector of cycads as well as rare and giant aloes. On his death the collection was presented to the Durban Botanic Gardens. A crane was even employed to lift and transport them to their new home!

Judith says:

My grandfather's garden was like a jungle: an everlasting source of wonder to me as a child. My mother inherited his love of plants and was a very gifted gardener. I grew up in a household where plants and medicine held sway. My father was a Scots GP, who despised the drug companies and their representatives and always talked of the importance of Nature in healing. In his day holistic medicine was still suspect. Were he alive today, he would have shown considerable interest in healing plants.

My first personal encounter with the marvellous healing properties of Aloe *vera* was in 1989. Bob Geldof had relaunched himself as a singer, following years of association with Live Aid. I was working for his manager at the time. One of his first London concerts was at the Town and Country Club. The day of the concert saw him huddled in a corner, suffering from a heavy cold and a croaking voice. At 2 o'clock that afternoon I gave him a strong dose of Aloe *vera*, plus some bee propolis. He shouted his familiar expletive at the bitterness of the juice! That evening he was able to perform with only the very slightest hint of huskiness in his voice.

My second encounter with the healing properties of Aloe *vera* was later that year with an outstanding Englishwoman who stayed with me as my guest. She had lived for 18 years in a cave in India, meditating high in the Himalayas, and had now returned to Britain. Years of living in a cold cave and enduring snowy winters at 13,200 feet had taken their toll and she suffered seriously from arthritis, to the point where it was extremely painful for her to walk even a few hundred yards. Her English name was Diane Perry; her adopted Tibetan name on becoming a mendicant nun was Tenzin Palmo.

As she was in so much pain, I gave her Aloe *vera* juice regularly. After a couple of months her condition had considerably improved. I continued to send her bottles of Aloe *vera* at her request once she returned to Italy. Combined with a careful diet, she is now free from arthritic suffering. Where she was once hardly able to walk up the street, she now travels and lectures worldwide, leading a very active life.

A strange and synchronous event occurred while writing this book. Dr Maikov had sent me a book from Moscow in Russian on Aloe *vera*. I asked a Russian friend, Natasha Hull (née Vassilieva) to translate the book orally for me. When I mentioned Professor Filatow and his pioneering work on Aloe therapy in Russia, she leapt up in amazement. 'You don't mean the great Filatow. My grandmother was his favourite student!' I am very grateful to Natasha for her invaluable help.

It is our wish that this book will prove useful and inspirational, and that people everywhere will be able to benefit from this truly remarkable plant.

Julia Lawless and Judith Allan
Hampstead, October 1999

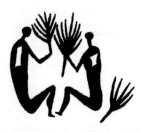

Aloe Vera

THE PLANT OF IMMORTALITY

Introduction:

The Aloe is a medicine recommended by the most respected tradition, it is used and affirmed by the experience of all doctors of all ages.

Dictionnaire Encyclopédique des Sciences Médicales, **Masson et Fils, Paris, 1865**

The use of Aloe *vera* will be the most important single step forward in the treatment of diseases in the history of mankind.

Dr McDaniel MD, Chief of Pathology, Dallas-Fort Worth Medical Center, Texas

Aloe *vera* is a remarkable plant ... one of a handful of traditional folk remedies renowned since ancient times as a 'cure all'. It has been called by such evocative names as 'Wand of Heaven', 'Miracle Worker' and 'Silent Healer', while the ancient Egyptians referred to it as 'The Plant of Immortality'. Indeed, one of the most outstanding qualities of Aloe *vera* is the versatile nature of its healing properties. Although it is best known today simply as a cosmetic ingredient, modern research is confirming the value of Aloe *vera* in the treatment of numerous disorders. These range from common complaints such as acne, eczema, indigestion and psoriasis to more serious medical conditions such as arthritis, ulcers, radiation burns, irritable bowel syndrome and even AIDS and cancer.

Aloe *vera* resembles a cactus with its characteristic spiky, fleshy leaves. In fact it is a perennial succulent belonging to the *Aloaceae* family. There are around 350 varieties of the Aloe plant, but the one with the best-known medicinal qualities is simply called Aloe *vera*, meaning the 'true aloe'. There are also four or five other varieties which are commonly used in healing.

The distinctive appearance of the Aloe *vera* plant is depicted on Egyptian temple friezes as early as 4000 BC, while its first recorded therapeutic use has been traced to a Sumerian clay tablet dated at around 2000 BC.

Although the medical versatility of the plant was known to early civilizations, and its usage documented by such prominent physicians as Dioscorides, Pliny the Elder and Galen, it was only early in the 20th century that its healing potential began to be re-assessed in the light of newly emerging scientific evidence. During the 1930s, in the pioneering days of x-ray treatment, it was found that Aloe *vera* juice could bring prompt healing to burns caused by radiation. When all other remedies failed, it also brought relief to victims of Hiroshima and Nagasaki who were severely burned.

Its more general usage was made possible in the late 1940s when a method to stop the oxidation and deterioration of the active ingredients in the plant was discovered. Subsequent tests confirmed that pain and scarring caused by burns and wounds was greatly reduced, if not entirely eradicated, due to a 'wound hormone'[1] contained in Aloe *vera*. Nowadays, Aloe *vera* extracts are used extensively in burn ointments, suntan lotions and skin care products.

During the 1980s and 1990s, further clinical studies have demonstrated that, apart from its cosmetic and skin care applications, Aloe *vera* promotes rapid healing and is also very effective as a natural painkiller, antibiotic, anti-inflammatory, immuno-stimulant and general antiseptic agent.

Some remarkable case histories and personal experiences of the benefits of Aloe *vera* can be found among people from all walks of life ... such accounts speak volumes about the healing capacity of this extraordinary plant.

Mahatma Gandhi drank Aloe *vera* juice every day. In a letter to his biographer, Romain Rolland, Gandhi wrote:

> You ask me what were the secret forces that sustained me during my long fasts. Well, it was my unshakeable faith in God, my simple and frugal lifestyle, and the Aloe whose benefits I discovered upon my arrival in South Africa at the end of the 19th century.

In 1995, Lady Elizabeth Anson, cousin to Queen Elizabeth II and an inveterate party-giver, revealed that it was Aloe *vera* which had given her a new lease of life after suffering from the debilitating effects of ME for many years. She has set up a charity for ME sufferers which recommends Aloe, among other natural treatments, to fellow sufferers.

Princess Helena Moutafian MBE, Dame of the Order of St John and a well-known humanitarian, uses Aloe *vera* daily. She uses the juice for eczema on her hands and face and takes Aloe *vera* capsules internally for bowel irritation and any kind of infection. In her view:

...Aloe is one of the best things that God created.

Dr David Smallbone, MB, CHB, LRCP, MRCS, MFHOM, FCOH, is a doctor and surgeon who has been in private practice in Britain since the late 1970s. He has not written a prescription for the last 10 to 15 years and now uses virtually no allopathic medicine. He treats his patients with a variety of natural methods such as herbal medicine and homoeopathy. Regarding Aloe *vera* he says:

> I have used Aloe *vera* in my practice over the years whenever I feel it to be necessary ... it is such a wonderful plant.

Stephen Turoff, one of the most gifted healers in Britain today, recommends Aloe as a general tonic and says that it is especially valuable in treating digestive disorders. In his view:

> Aloe *vera* is good for everything...

Botanical, Historical and Cultural Origins

PART ONE

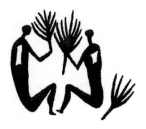

The Aloe Vera Family Tree

ALOE VERA

Most sources place Aloe in the Lily family (*Liliaceae*). Until recently this was correct, but according to Dr Tom Reynolds of the Jodrell Laboratory, Kew Gardens, London, it has now been designated its own family, known as *Aloaceae*. Nonetheless, it is related to the lily family and to plants such as garlic, onion and asparagus, all of which are known to have medicinal properties.

The Royal Horticultural Society Gardeners' Encylopaedia of Plants and Flowers defines Aloe as:

> [A] Genus of evergreen, rosetted trees, shrubs, perennials and scandent climbers with succulent foliage and tubular to bell-shaped flowers.[1]

There are about 350 varieties of Aloe in the *Aloaceae* family. In South Africa alone, 132 species were recorded in 1955! They range from miniature aloes like Aloe *aristata* and Aloe *brevifolia* to small aloes such as Aloe *striata*, which is one of the prettiest of the species. Its leaves are pale green edged with light coral red and sometimes flushed with pink. The flowers are orange or pinky-red and roughly resemble a mass of coral. The flowers of different aloes vary in colour from cream or orange to scarlet, rose flame or spectacular autumn tints.

Among the large aloes are Aloe *arborescens* and Aloe *ferox*, both used for healing purposes. In the 19th century, James Backhouse, in *A Narrative of a Visit to Mauritius and South Africa*, refers to Aloe *arborescens* as a Tree-Aloe, otherwise known as 'Kokerboom' in the Afrikaans language. 'Kokerboom' means Quiver Tree, as it was used by the Bushmen to make quivers from its branches. Members of the *Aloaceae* family known for their medicinal properties include:

- Aloe *arborescens*, which is used in Japan and has been cultivated mainly in Russia and the Far East. It has long slender blue-green leaves with toothed edges, and cream stripes. It produces numerous spikes of red flowers in late winter and spring, and grows to a height of 1.8 m (6 ft) high.

- Aloe *ferox* or Aloe *ferox* 'Miller' has a red or reddish pink flower and has been identified as being the same plant as Aloe *african* 'Miller'. Its flowers are described as orange-scarlet according to the Royal Horticultural Society. This Aloe originated in South Africa and is also referred to as the Cape Aloe. This only adds to the confusion, as in southern Africa Aloe *barbadensis* 'Miller' is known as the Cape Aloe. Nor is Aloe *african* 'Miller' the same plant as Aloe *africana*. Aloe *africana* has a yellow flower. It is not the same species and is not officially recognized as being a medicinal source.

- Aloe *perryi* 'Baker' is otherwise known as the Socotrine or Curaçaon Aloe, after the islands of Socotra and Curaçao where it is found. Other names include Zanzibar Aloes, Uganda Aloes,

Natal Aloes and Musambra Aloes. The flowers of Aloe *perryi* 'Baker' are bright red with a greenish tip.

- Aloe *saponaria*, found all over South Africa, Swaziland and Zimbabwe, is one of the spotted Aloes, with dull white oblong spots on its leaves. The flowers are orangey-yellow in colour.

- Aloe *vera* (L.) Burm.f is the correct name for Aloe *vera*, which was formerly known as Aloe *barbadensis* 'Miller'. According to Dr Tom Reynolds of Kew Gardens, 'Burman had priority over Miller's later use of the name A. *barbadensis*, but perhaps only be a period of 10 days ... the correct name is thus Aloe *vera* (L.) Burm.f.'[2] It is considered very effective in healing and is characterized by its very sticky mucilage.

The origins of Aloe *vera* is not clearly known. Some writers claim it comes from southern Africa, others from northern Africa. One of the most authoritative botanical sources, Mr Nigel Hepper, retired senior botanist at Kew Gardens, has suggested that it may come from the Yemen. This has not been proven, but the Aloe *vera* plant has been found in the Yemen in remote places where it was clearly not transplanted from another region. It has also been found in Tenerife in mountainous areas. In the light of early Egyptian and Mesopotamian records, it most likely comes from either the Yemen or North Africa.

Aloe *vera* is a clump-forming, perennial succulent with basal rosettes of tapering, thick leaves, mottled green, later turning grey-green. It is a cactus-like plant with distinctive spiky leaves whose flower stems carry bell-shaped yellow flowers in summer. From the centre of the dark green leaves of the Aloe *vera* plant, the flower stems, which are leafless, can reach 1.5 m (3 ft) in length and have attractive tubular-shaped bells.

The Aloe *vera* plant is characterized by its long tapering sharp leaves with ribbed thorny ridges along the spine. The fleshy leaves grow in a spiral shape to form a rosette pattern. This rosette pattern is a distinctive feature of Aloe *vera*. The soft fleshy leaves of the Aloe *vera* exude a watery gel or juice when cut, and contain the plant's two main medicinal products:

> 1 the sap from the rind, known as the exudate
>
> 2 the gel/juice, used extensively in healing.

The leaves themselves can also be dried and made into powder (for use in beauty products). All medical aloes, however, produce a typical bitter yellowish or reddish sap which is their common characteristic.

All Aloes are part of a larger genus called Xeroids, which implies an ability to 'shut down' the pores (or 'stomata', tiny openings in the epidermis of the leaf) to ensure that water is retained within the plant. In this way they can survive long periods without water. This same ability to close the stomata in the leaf also apparently facilitates the almost miraculous closing of any wound or damage to the outer skin of the plant. The power to heal itself so rapidly and re-grow in another direction doubtless pointed the way to its use as a wound treatment.

The Aloe *vera* plant takes about four years to mature, by which time the gel in the outer leaves is at its most potent. When fully grown the individual leaves can reach a height of 60 to 90 cm (2 to 3 ft) and each leaf can weigh approximately 1.5 to 2 kg (3 to 4 lb). Each plant usually has 12 to 16 leaves. As a perennial, Aloe *vera* lives for about 12 years. When the outer leaves are harvested, up to three times a year, the plant is able to close itself down against water loss. Within a few seconds of being cut, the plant films over the wound and a protective coating forms which stops loss of sap. The outer leaves are always harvested first, allowing the inner leaves time to develop their ripeness and potency.

Although Aloe is ideally suited to growing in hot, arid climates, it can be grown in glasshouses or indoors in Europe. As it is frost-sensitive it should always be kept in warm conditions, requiring a minimum temperature of 7–10°C (45–50°F). However, although frost can kill them, the plants seldom die simply from exposure to cold unless they are very young. Tree Aloes and shrubs with a spread over 30 cm (1 ft) prefer full sun; most smaller species require partial shade. The plant also requires very well-drained soil. Ideally, in warmer climates it likes sun for at least two hours a day, porous or sandy soil and exposure to the wind. The wind actually conditions and strengthens the thick meaty leaves.

The Aloe is easily propagated since at the base of the plant, suckers or 'pups' grow which can be separated to make new cuttings. Apart from their requirement for warmth, an Aloe *vera* plant is very easy to maintain as a house plant or conservatory specimen. Watering should be infrequent and less so during winter months. Like orchids, Aloes can be killed by too much care and water!

Myth, Legend and Folklore

ALOE VERA

Aloe *vera* has been in use for over 5,000 years. Throughout the ages it has maintained its reputation as being a seemingly magical plant, able to cure all or almost all ailments. As such, it is natural that it has given birth to a plethora of legendary tales, some which have their root in fact while others belong to the realm of myth.

The Early Egyptians, Hebrews and Greeks

Known as the 'Plant of Immortality' by the early Egyptians, there are tales that Aloe was used in the embalming process and also in the burial rites of the Pharaohs. In addition, the beauty of Nefertiti and Cleopatra was attributed to the use of Aloe. Cleopatra apparently owed her extraordinary good looks to bathing in a mixture of Aloe gel and goat's milk. Aloe, finely powdered, was also said to have been used to make her eyes bright in the same way we use eyebright nowadays. The Pharaohs believed that the plant had magic powers and assigned it a royal status within their household.

As for its uses in embalming, it might well be that Aloe is being confused with aloeswood, Lignum (or Lignin) Aloes, from the East African Aloes tree (*Aquilaria agallocha*). The oil from Lignum aloes was used by the Hebrews to perfume their beds, anoint their bodies and cover the smell of decaying flesh during the burial ceremony. The same myth persists in Biblical references which claim that Aloe was used in the embalming of Christ:

> And there came also, Nicodemus, which at the first came Jesus by night, and brought a mixture of myrrh and aloes, about a hundred pounds weight ... Then they took the body of Jesus and wound it in linen cloth with the spices, as the manner of the Jews is to bury. [John 19:39–40]

One of the earliest and most popular surviving legends is that Alexander the Great, after his conquest of Persia in 333 BC, was persuaded by his tutor Aristotle to conquer the island of Socotra in order to obtain Aloe plants. Socotra lies off the east coast of Africa between Aden and Somalia. It is said that Alexander drove the inhabitants off the island and used the plant in his military campaigns, as a healing balm for his soldiers' wounds. This Aloe was known as Aloe *succotrina*, which is one of the earliest classifications of Aloe *vera*. Reputedly there were five Aloe *vera* plantations on Socotra, which apparently traded with China, India, Tibet and Malaysia. It is questionable indeed whether Alexander actually engaged in such a conquest, as records suggest that this island lies 1,500 miles south of Alexander's known conquests.

Eastern Cultures

Claims that Aloe *vera* was taken into Tibet from Socotra also appear to be unsubstantiated in Tibetan medicine. Popular references denote Aloe as 'jelly leeks' in Tibet. The only reference to 'jelly leeks' being used in areas close to Tibet is in 1943 by Colonel M Thomas Tchou of Tzechow, which lies in Western China at the foothills of the Himalayas. In 1901 he used Aloe gel on a burnt hand, as recommended by his aunt. His sores healed. Some 38 years later Tchou met a Dr Cole in Cleveland, Ohio, who advised him to use Aloe *vera* to treat ulceration caused by radiation. Immediately Tchou then recognized that it was the same plant his aunt had given him so many years before in China.

While Aloe *vera* was used in India and China, it is possible that what was referred to in Tibet was aloeswood, which is used for the making of incense or medicine. In Ayurvedic medicine, aloeswood (*Aquilaria agallocha*) is known in Hindi as *Agar* and in Sanskrit as *Agaru*; Tibetan medicine employs *Agar* as a treatment for hyper-activity and to induce restful sleep. Chronicler Ain-i-Abari reported during the reign of the Moghul Emperor Akbar (about 1595) that 'Aloeswood is often used in compound perfumes. When eaten, it is exhilarating. It is generally employed in incense. The better qualities, powdered, are used for rubbing into the skin and clothes.'[1] *Agar* forms the Indian word for incense – *agarbati*, or 'lighted aloeswood'. In Ayurvedic medicine the powdered wood of the Aloe tree is used as a skin tonic and as a gentle antiseptic for ear and eye infections, as well as for open wounds. These medical uses could easily provide an explanation for the confusion with Aloe *vera*.

Aphrodisiac qualities are also attributed to Aloe in the classical Indian guide to sexuality, the Kama Sutra. In China too, Aloe *vera* has been traditionally mixed with liquorice to be drunk as a tonic. These cultures believed that Aloe *vera* possessed magical properties conducive to good health, happiness, sexual prowess and long life. Like the Chinese who drank Aloe *vera* to enhance their sexual prowess, the Roman Emperor Tiberius purportedly drank Aloe *vera* juice to increase his potency! Thousands of miles away, the native American Navajos also extolled its energizing sexual qualities, as did members of certain South American tribes. Although it is easy to exaggerate these claims, contemporary studies in sexuality have shown that there is a close link between levels of virility and nutrition. Since Aloe *vera* is extremely rich in nutrients, this is not such an unlikely or unfounded use for the plant. Furthermore, the Russians have been using Aloe successfully to treat male impotence (see First Aid section, page 137).

The New World

In the popular imagination, Christopher Columbus has also been traditionally linked with Aloe *vera*. Perhaps the best known of all these 'legends' is that Columbus carried Aloe *vera* plants on his first voyage to the New World. This was because he wanted to use it as a treatment for sunburns, cuts, wounds and other accidents liable to occur on board ship. Although Aloes are mentioned twice in his logs of 1492, there is some doubt as to what plant Columbus was referring. In fact it is more likely he was carrying the Agave plant, which has also been used for healing purposes and which is easily mistaken for Aloe *vera* by the uninitiated. At that period Aloe *vera* was not known to exist in Northern America except in Florida, Texas and California. There are, however, other records which suggest that Columbus documented the presence of Aloe in Cuba and other Caribbean islands.

Ponce de Leon, the 15th-century Spanish explorer, went to America in search of 'the fountain of youth'. The native Seminole people of Florida showed him

Aloe and its many uses, including its benefits as a digestive aid, hair-restorer and life-giving tonic. According to the native Americans, the elixir of long life resided in a pool in the middle of a cluster of Aloe *vera* leaves!

An Aloe by Any Other Name...

Aloe is known throughout many cultures by different poetic names, many of which reflect its legendary association with immortality. The origin of the word is generally traced to the Arabic word 'alloeh' which means 'bitter and shiny substance'. There are other possible sources, but this seems to be the most plausible. As the ancients used either the sap or the ground leaf, in both instances the result is a shiny and bitter substance. In Hebrew it is referred to as 'halal' (or 'allal' – bitter) which means 'shiny bitter substance', as does the Syrian name for it, 'alwai'. In ancient Hebrew it was called 'ahaloth'.

The ancient Chinese considered the plant to have major therapeutic qualities and called it the 'Harmonic Remedy'. In 9th-century China, the leaves were said to look like the 'tail of a giant crab'. Chinese Materia Medica refer to Aloe *vera* either as Aloe *chinensis* or Aloe *vulgaris*. Knowledge of the plant seemed to be predominantly in the province of Canton, as it entered China through the trading port of Canton. It was 'much used in the worm-fever and convulsions of children' and for skin infections, mixed with liquorice.[2] The Chinese referred to the plant as having come from Persia, Java and Sumatra. In 1985, in a contemporary Chinese herbal, Him-che Yeung refers to Aloe *vera* as having anti-cancer properties, anti-fungal and anti-parasitic properties as well as it being a purgative and wound healer.

In Ayurvedic medicine Aloe *vera* is known as 'Ghrita-Kumari': 'Kumari' means a young girl, virgin or a maiden, and Aloe was so-called because it brings about the renewal of female energy and imparts the energy of youth. In Ayurvedic medicine, the gel is used as one of the most important tonics for the female reproductive system, the liver and for regulating fire. The gel can be used for premenstrual tension, regulating menstrual flow, menopause and for women who have had hysterectomies. In Ayurveda, it is considered good for all three 'humours' or 'constitutional types': Vata (characterized by nervousness and sensitivity), Pitta (fiery), and Kapha (steady, regular, prone to sluggishness).

The Arabs called it the 'Desert Lily'. The Knights Templar, who drank a heady mixture of palm wine, aloe pulp and hemp, called it the 'Elixir of Jerusalem', attributing their longevity and health to it.

In Japan Aloe *vera* is popularly called 'No Need of a Doctor'; in Java it is known as 'Crocodile's Tongue', and in Malaysia as 'Mother-in-law's tongue' – no doubt referring to its bitter taste and the pointed sharp leaves! Infinitely more poetic is 'The Wand of Heaven' as it was known in Egypt. Elsewhere it has been called 'Heaven's blessing plant', the 'Mystical plant' or 'Miracle plant', the 'Magic medicine plant' and the 'Flow of Life'. It is more accurately known as the 'Burn plant' in current terminology or the 'First Aid plant', 'Wound-healing plant' and 'Man's natural medicine chest'. In contemporary America it is known as 'the Silent Healer'.

Like the Egyptians, the native Seminole people of Florida, and native Mexicans, call Aloe *vera* the 'Plant of Immortality'. The Russians echo the ancient Egyptians' praise of Aloe *vera* by calling it the 'Elixir of Longevity'. So revered and beloved has this plant been throughout different cultures and periods in our history that the list of names goes on and on, all praising Aloe *vera*'s qualities in a practical or poetic fashion.

The Elixir of Longevity

The claim to Aloe being an aid to longevity was borne out by an extraordinary Frenchman in the last century, a philosopher and a practitioner of medicine, a man administering to the poor in the belief that medicines should not be prohibitive, nor health the privilege of the rich:

> During the 20 years that I have been treating my patients with Aloe, I have found that there are many diseases described by the doctors of antiquity which disappear rapidly when I administer Aloe in the form of granules or powder. Therefore, the good results which I have always obtained allow me to quote the adage of Roger Bacon: 'Do you wish to live as long as Noah? Then take some pills of Aloah!'[3]
>
> **François Vincent Raspail (1794–1878)**

In a more profound sense, Aloe *vera*'s symbolic association with long life and immortality, its association with embalming and the transition between one life and the next, may lie in the renewing nature of the plant itself. J Norris in the *Garden Journal* (New York Botanical Garden, 1973) wrote:

If a plant is able to heal its own wounds, to survive without nourishment, even seemingly to return from the dead, might not its power somehow be applicable to man's own maladies?[4]

Traditional Uses

Aloe has appeared in all the most advanced Materia Medica of the great ancient civilizations: Egypt, Mesopotamia, Arabia, Greece, Rome as well as in China and India. These civilizations were trustees of knowledge concerning the healing powers of Aloe *vera*, a knowledge which they passed on to their successors living around the Mediterranean region and subsequently to the whole of the Western world. They in turn traded with Africa, where the majority of Aloes have originated: thus the story of Aloe goes full circle...

Africa is the source of many varieties of the Aloe plant, and so it is natural that it features strongly in the ethnographic lore of both the North and South. A number of tribal uses for the plant have been documented, and anthropologists report on the widespread use of Aloe among the tribes of southern Africa – the Zulus, the Sutos and the Xhosa being the best known. The Aloes used vary regionally and are not popularly known except for Aloe *ferox*; Aloe *macracantha*; Aloe *tenuior Haw.*, Aloe *marlothii A. Berg* and Aloe *variegata L.*, are among those that have been used traditionally.

The Sutos tribes use Aloe as a natural antiseptic. When colds or influenza become a threatening epidemic, a public bath infused with Aloe is taken by the villagers. The plant is used as protection against lightning, by sprinkling burnt, crushed and boiled bits of the plant around the village. Barren Suto women drink a concoction from Aloe juice to aid their fertility. Nor is its use limited to tribe-members alone. If their animals are wounded, ash from the burnt leaves of Aloe is placed on the ground beneath the injured limb to hasten healing.

The fresh juice from the Aloe leaf is used by the Sutos, Zulus and Xhosa to treat eye infections, applied directly to the eye. In the Transvaal, an Aloe *variegata* infusion in brandy is used to treat haemorrhoids.

The Zulu women in South Africa use Aloe to help wean their babies, by spreading the bitter gel on their breasts. A decoction of the Aloe *arborescens* leaf is given to Zulu women just before they give birth, to aid the birth process. (In the Transvaal, a vinous extract of Aloe *sp.* is used for abortive purposes). The Zulus also use the plant, steeped in water, as an enema to clean out the intestines. Even the flowers of the plant are not wasted. Ground up into powder, which is then steeped in water, it is used to treat feverish colds in children, either orally or as an enema. The flowers are also cooked by the Zulus and eaten. It is good for snuff: tobacco is mixed with the ash of the Aloe leaf. In addition, Aloe has traditionally been used in South Africa as a cure for venereal diseases.[1]

In general, a number of southern African tribes use Aloe for stomach problems. They drink 'a decoction of the roots' which can cause vomiting if taken in large amounts.[2]

The Xhosas and other tribes use Aloe to treat tape worm infection. It is considered effective with no side-effects. Both the gel and juice are used in the treatment of ringworm. It is also used as a purgative, a treatment for boils and sores. It is said that Xhosa children are fond of sucking the nectar-like juice out of the flowers, which is said to create weakness in the joints if taken over a long period. It also has a narcotic effect!

The southern African tribes use Aloe with their animals, in the treatment of scab with sheep and as a purgative. Aloe *saponaria Haw.*, known as 'White-spotted aloe' or 'Soap aloe', is used in the treatment of 'blood scours' in calves and to treat indigestion and enteritis in fowls, both with excellent results. The Zulus believe that the smoke from burning leaves of Aloe protects cattle from the ill-effects of eating the wrong food.

In Africa and the East, the plant was even said to have been used to ward off evil spirits. Hung over the entrance to a house, it ensured a long life for its inhabitants. It could also be worn as an amulet around the neck to guarantee a happy and healthy life.

Richard Burton, the 19th-century explorer and naturalist, reported on his African travels that Aloe *vera*, suspended above one's bed, was effective against mosquitoes. In Columbia the live plant is used in shops to repel flies and the juice is rubbed on children's legs to protect them from insect bites. Recent research has shown Aloe *vera* to be an effective insect-repellent by virtue of its bitter taste and the unpleasant smell of the sap.

Aloes were depicted in rock paintings by the Bushmen in the early 18th century, according to Miss D F Bleek in her book, *Rock Paintings in South Africa*. These rock paintings were found near the Orange River in the Orange Free State, in a cave by a waterfall. Miss Bleek suggests that the Aloes depicted are Aloe *ferox* 'Miller' and Aloe *broomii*. Walter Battiss in his *The Artists of the Rocks* (1948) suggests that this 'painting of Aloes is a most remarkable painting in the whole of the art. It belongs to the Last Period of Bushman Art.'[3] The Aloes are shown clasped in the Bushmen's hands like triumphal candelabras, two figures facing each other. Another figure holds it in his hand pointed to the earth, while another Bushman lies prostrate below a floating aloe. Two other Bushmen are shown hunting with large dominant buck, possibly antelope, behind them. This suggests that Aloes were an integral part of life and nourishment in the Bush, as important as hunting for survival. The juice of Aloe *saponaria* is still used by hunters in the Congo, in Central Africa, who smear their body with it before the hunt. The bitter smell of the Aloe juice masks the hunter's smell and blocks perspiration, thus making the hunter more invisible to his prey. Aloe *saponaria* is also used in Southern Africa for healing battle or hunting wounds.

In the 9th century AD, Al-Kindi of Baghdad wrote *The Medical Formulary*, also known as 'the Aqrabadhin of Al-Kindi'. Al-Kindi was known as the 'philosopher of Arabia'. In *The Medical Formulary* he makes several references to the use of Aloe, particularly in relation to eye treatments. In all remedies, Aloe is mixed with other ingredients – for example, gold, red hematite and saffron, or myrrh and saffron along with soapwort, sweet marjoram and lycium juice – then pulverized and kneaded and made into pills. When required, the pills are dissolved in woman's milk and oil of violet before being used. His remedies nearly always end with 'It is good and effective with God's help.'[4]

Al-Kindi records that the Arabs called Aloe *vera sabir* or *sabr*, while the Syrians called the plant *sabhra* or *sebara*. There is a valley in Lebanon known as the Sabhra Valley, which translates as the Valley of the Aloes. The two languages are similar and the meaning is the same in all cases – 'bitter and shiny substance'.

Aloe was, as ever, a well known purgative, but Al-Kindi also noted its anti-inflammatory action, its effective opthalmological uses (such as its effectiveness with eye ulcers) and its positive action as regarded melancholia. It was also helpful with *dyspnoea* or difficult breathing. As a purgative drug, Aloe was treated with caution. Aloe was also being used throughout the Middle East: in the lands around the Red Sea, Aloe *latifolia* was believed to cure both ringworm and impetigal infections.

A note of caution came from the mediaeval medical writer Mesue of Damascus, who gave a rather graphic report of side-effects which even included piles. One lurid story concerned Emperor Otto II, who took too much Aloe and died in AD 983.[5]

It is generally held that it was Arab traders who first brought Aloe *vera* to Persia and India about the 6th century BC. According to Chopra's 'Indigenous Drugs of India', Aloe was already widely used in India during Hippocrates' lifetime (460–375 BC), and its medicinal uses dated 'back to the 4th century BC'.[6] Early medical texts from India indicate its use for skin inflammations. A Portugese naturalist, Garcia da Orta, later described the Hindus using Aloe *vera* for 'purgatives, in kidney disease, colic, and also for healing wounds', including the treatment of eye sores.[7] Aloe *vera* still plays an important role in the traditional medicine of India, where Aloe *vera* preparations are particularly important for their cathartic (purgative or laxative), stomachic (digestive), emmenagogic (aiding in menstruation) and anthelmintic (expelling intestinal worms) properties. In addition, Aloe *vera* gel is considered one of the most important tonics for the female reproductive system, the liver, heart and spleen.

From India, the use of Aloe *vera* probably spread to Java, Malaysia, Sumatra and to the rest of the East Indies. In Java it was applied as skin care on infections, sunburn and blisters, while Aloe *barbadensis* was taken internally for gonorrheal infections. In addition it was used internally for tuberculosis in much the same way as it was in Europe: as a popular cure for consumption. In Malaya, Aloe *vera* pulp was bound onto the forehead to relieve headaches; in the Philippines it was used to reduce swelling (oedema) in beri-beri sufferers. As in Europe, when mixed with wine it was considered effective in preventing hair loss. In the East Indies there are reports that Aloe *vera* was popular for treating conditions such as gout, or aches and pains in the joints and bones.

The same conditions were traditionally treated with Aloe in the Caribbean. It was used for skin care and to treat problems such as cuts, blisters, wounds and insect bites. Its use in internal ailments appears to have been taught by the missionaries and explorers. In the Caribbean today it is still used for both human and animal ailments. Apparently the leaf is sucked as though it were sugar cane! Aloe *vera* juice, fed to horses, makes the horses' blood so bitter that ticks apparently fall off after the first bite! It is also used for delousing, repelling infestations and as a life-giving tonic during cattle birth trauma.

From India and the East Indies, the use of Aloe spread into the Canton province in China. No doubt it was also brought to China by Arab traders. Chinese medical texts refer to Aloe from the 7th century AD onwards; the first noted use was for healing dermatitis. Aloe *vera* was especially noted for its use as a treatment for sinusitis and worm fever, as well as for convulsions in children and skin afflictions such as eczema.

The Venetian Marco Polo, travelling through China in the 13th century, found Aloe *vera* was used to treat rashes and other skin disorders, as well as for stomach ailments. Today, although Aloe *chinensis* is one of the best known regional variations of the healing Aloes, Aloe *arborescens* is used to treat burns in China and Russia. In addition, Aloe *arborescens* has been used in Japan as a folk remedy for burns, insect bites, wound-healing, athlete's foot and digestive complaints. In his *Il Milione*, Polo documents Aloe's history and legend, tracing its development and usage from the Island of Socotra through to the Orient, via the great Eastern trading routes.

Wound-healer

Aloe *vera*'s use as a wound-healer and for general skin treatment is perhaps its most universally acclaimed virtue among many diverse and distant ethnic groups. In northern Mexico and the Rio Grande Valley of South Texas, Aloe *vera*, known as *savila*, grows profusely and is used to heal skin diseases. In Mexico the leaves are gathered in the semi-wild to treat burns, bruises, skin irritations and even leprosy. In Florida, Aloe *vera* is widespread and has been used traditionally for treating jelly-fish stings as well as bee stings. Mayan women in the Yucatan region of Mexico have used Aloe *vera* for centuries to moisturize their skin. Like the Zulus in southern Africa, they also use it to wean their children from breast-feeding.

Throughout Central and South America, the pulp of Aloe *vera* is regarded as a mild laxative; another one of its earliest and most common uses worldwide. Indeed, the early Arabs' principal use of the drug Aloes was as a laxative, although other uses were suggested in Persian records of the 6th century BC. They were using it both internally and externally, and processed the plant by separating the gel and sap from the rind using their bare feet. The resulting pulp was placed in goatskin bags and dried in the sun before the contents were ground into powder. Still today Aloe is called the 'Desert Lily' by the Bedouin tribes and the Tuareg of the Sahara Desert.

The Age of Discovery

ALOE VERA

A Sumerian clay tablet, found in the city of Nippur in Mesopotamia and dating from around 2,000 BC, includes Aloe in its list of useful healing plants. This is the earliest recorded pharmaceutical use of Aloe and predates the written Egyptian records, which are commonly cited as being the first known source of Aloe *vera* and its medicinal uses.

Around 1500 BC, during the reign of the Pharaoh Amen-Hotep I, the Egyptians gave us the first detailed analysis of Aloe's medical value in the Papyrus Ebers.[1] This was named after the German Egyptologist Georg Ebers who, together with a wealthy German called Herr Gunther, bought it in the winter of 1872 from an Egyptian who had found it in 1858 between the knees of a mummy in a tomb at El Assassif, near Thebes. The Papyrus Ebers was given intact to the University of Leipzig, where it remains to this day in almost perfect condition.

The Papyrus Ebers is not so much a coherent text as a collection of medical documents and folklore on the causes and treatments of diseases and the correct religious rites to accompany them. Ebers considered the book to be one of the 'Hermetic Books' of the ancient Egyptians. It is the earliest known complete papyrus extant, and is extremely detailed. In fact it is a miscellaneous collection compiled from at least 40 different sources. Some of the material is much older than 1500 BC, anything from 500 or 2,000 years prior to the date it became a coherent text.

In ancient Egypt, medicine and healing were intricately connected with the spiritual life: incantations were used to invoke those gods who ruled life and healing, in particular Isis and Ra. Uses for Aloe were both pharmaceutical and spiritual.

Although it is customary to refer to the Papyrus Ebers as giving 12 formulae for the use of Aloe to treat a number of disorders, this is now questionable following consultation with the Egyptian Department of the British Museum. According to Miss Carol Andrews, Assistant Keeper of Egyptian Antiquities, on checking two-thirds of the remedies we find that only two refer to a plant which has a bitter, disagreeable taste and needs to be compensated for with the sweetness of honey. It would appear that this is Aloe *vera*. The other remedies refer to cinnamon bark, which could have been confused with aloeswood, another aromatic wood.

Greek doctors did some of their medical training in the great school of Alexandria and their knowledge of the Aloe plant surpassed that of the Egyptians. Aloe was first mentioned in Greek pharmacology by Celsius (25 BC–AD 50) when it was referred to as a purgative, one of the best known and earliest uses of the plant. It is to a famous 1st-century Greek physician, Pedanius Dioscorides of Anazarba, however, that we are indebted for his extensive work on the plant in his *De Materia Medica* (AD 41–68). This is the first detailed Western treatise following on from the Papyrus Ebers and describes more than 600 plants.

Some 400 years later, the Greek *Herbal* of Dioscorides was illustrated by a Byzantine and called the *Codex Anicine Julianae*. It is found in Vienna and includes some of the oldest surviving representations of Eastern Mediterranean plants, including a coloured plate of Aloe *vera*.

It took a further 1,500 years from the time of Dioscorides before his *De Materia Medica* was translated into English by John Goodyer. From this 15th-century translation, together with knowledge of the works of Pliny the Elder (AD 23–79), the great classical physician Rufus of Ephesus (early 2nd century AD) and the great Galen (late 2nd century AD), known as the Father of Modern Medicine, Western physicians learned of the wide range of Aloe's medical versatility. This included treating ulcerated genitals, healing the foreskin, getting rid of haemorrhoids, wound healing, treating insomnia and stomach disorders, reversing hair loss, treating mouth and gum diseases, boils, sunburn, constipation and kidney ailments. In addition, it prevented vomiting of blood, was an effective purgative and was good for tonsillitis and eye infections.

In an altogether charming description of the plant and its medicinal uses, Dioscorides describes the plant as having a leaf...

> like Squill, thick, gross, somewhat broad in ye compass, broken or bowbacked behind, but on either part it hath ye leaves prickly by ye sides, appearing thinly, short. But it sends out a stalk like to Anthericum, but a white flower, & a seed like until Asphodelus. All of it, is of a strong scent, & very bitter to ye taster, but it is but of one root having a root as a stake. It grows in India very much, gross, from

whence also ye extracted juice is brought. It grows also in Arabia and Asia, & in certain sea-bordering places and Islands, as in Andros, not good for extracting juice but fitting for ye conglutinating of wounds, being laid on when it is beaten small ...[2]

Medically Aloe's properties were wide-ranging, and Dioscorides recommended it for numerous conditions including:

> ...splitting of blood ... cleanseth ye Icterus ... taken either with water, or sod honey it looseth ye belly ... it assuageth Scabritias and the itchings of ye eye corner, and ye headache being anointed with acetum & Rosaceum, on ye forehead & the temples, & with wine it stays ye hair falling off, & with honey and wine it is good for ye tonsillae, as also the gums and all griefs in ye mouth. But it is roasted also for eye medicines in a cleane and red hot earthen vessell, being kept turned with a splatter until that it is roasted equally ...[3]

In the same period, Pliny the Elder (AD 23–79), a highly respected Roman physician, in his *Natural History* not only confirmed Dioscorides' writings on Aloes but also added his own medical findings. He advises that the best aloes to use 'will be fatty and shiny, of a ruddy colour, friable, compact like liver, and easily melted'. Aloe's nature is 'bracing, astringent and gently warming'. Of its many uses, the chief is to 'relax the bowels, for it is almost the only laxative that is also a stomach tonic, no ill effects whatever resulting from its use'. To regularize the bowels, he recommends Aloe in warm or cold water, taken two or three times daily as required. For hair loss prevention, Aloe mixed with dry wine should be rubbed on the head 'in the contrary way to the hair'. Mixed with rose oil and vinegar, Aloe soothed headaches if applied to the temples or forehead.[4]

Pliny discovered that the root of the Aloe could be boiled down and used as a treatment in leprosy, for healing leprous sores. Furthermore, he found that it could help check perspiration by mixing Aloe with rue boiled in rose oil. Doubtless this was the world's first-known anti-perspirant!

After Dioscorides and Pliny, it was the Greek physician Galen who dominated medical history from the 2nd century AD until the Middle Ages. In the earlier part of the 2nd century AD his predecessor, the great classical physician Rufus of Ephesus wrote *On the Interrogation of the Patient*. Galen often quotes Rufus of Ephesus in his own work. Both physicians studied anatomy at Alexandria.

Rufus of Ephesus used Aloe to treat various illnesses such as glaucoma, cataracts, melancholy and the plague. He also recommends its use in poor digestion and constipation, and points out that it modifies the secretion of bile, slows haemorrhages and is effective against 'rebellious ulcers'.[5]

Around the 2nd century AD extensive work was carried out by an unknown Syriac physician, probably a Nestorian, who studied medicine in Alexandria and compiled an extensive Materia Medica called *The Book of Medicines* (also known as *Syrian Anatomy, Pathology and Therapeutics*). This physician was clearly a learned and distinguished man, a follower of Hippocrates who wrote clearly and simply. He drew strongly on Dioscorides' work and the Papyrus

Ebers. Some of the text was written originally in Greek and the first section is a series of lectures, to which is added the most detailed prescriptions, one of which is known as the Pills of Galen.

This remarkable work contains some of the most extensive early remedies using Aloe in medicine, and are too numerous to mention here in detail. They range from Aloe being used as a purgative to treating eye, ear and throat infections, stomach disorders, haemorrhaging, chest infection, liver and spleen diseases, menstrual disorders, inflammation, paralysis, pain and abscesses. Aloe is used in combination with a number of other ingredients.

By the end of the 2nd century AD, the plant then had become an established part of the European pharmacopoeia. Not only Galen but also other physicians such as Antyllus, Aretacus and others purported to use Aloe in their healing repertoire. It is recognized that the period between the time of Hippocrates and that of Galen heralds one of the biggest advances in European medicine, covering a period of 500 to 600 years.

It was largely thanks to the Jesuit priests of Spain that the use of Aloe spread throughout the Western world during the 15th and 16th centuries. The Jesuits were highly educated physicians and scholars and their knowledge of the classics was unsurpassed. They were familiar with the Greek and Roman medical texts and therefore were fully conversant with the medicinal and pharmacological properties of the Aloe plant. Furthermore, the Jesuit Fathers were ever practical. As Aloe grew with such ease in Spain and Portugal, they simply took the plant along with them as they accompanied explorers on their colonial expeditions, and planted it wherever they settled. It was an extremely useful plant as it was so hardy and adaptable. If Aloe did not grow locally, they planted it. Such was the high esteem in which they held the plant.

In this way, Aloe was transported to places as far afield as Jamaica, Haiti, Antigua, South and Central America through the spread of missionary establishments. It settled easily into hot semi-tropical climates, and was also grown on plantations by traders aware of its medicinal and commercial value for the European market. In some areas where it grew naturally, like Curaçao and Florida, the Jesuit priests expanded local knowledge of its medicinal uses by drawing on their classical understanding.

With the conquest of the Aztec empire by the Spaniards, the missionaries introduced their knowledge of the healing plant to the Indians of Central America and Mexico.

Aloe was introduced into the island of Barbados at the end of the 16th century (1596), probably by the Jesuits, or possibly by African slaves. It is this Aloe which bears the name Aloe *barbadensis*, formerly the accepted nomenclature for Aloe *vera*. Here, the commercial plantations of Aloe turned into a major industry for the medical market.

As the Jesuits had spread Aloe *vera* throughout the New World, and rumour has it that this was as far afield as the Philippines, so it was the Dutch who capitalized on the use of Aloe for medicinal purposes in Africa. Before the end of the 17th century, the Aloe had already been taken back to Holland by Dutch traders, and Cape Aloes were being cultivated in some of Europe's finest gardens. At the Cape of Good Hope, Dutch colonists had laid out a garden for weary voyagers en route to India or China. The Jesuit Father Guy

Tachard wrote in 1685 that this was one of the 'most beautiful and curious gardens' he had ever seen.[6] It included at least 20 varieties of Aloe. It was nearly 100 years later that the British took to importing Aloe sap from South Africa.

In the colonial rush to acquire good natural resources for medical plants, Britain undoubtedly was eclipsed by both Spain and Holland. Instead, it looked to the British colony of Georgia, now an American state, for medicinal plants. An Apothecaries Company had been set up with the aim of supplying drugs and other materials to Britain. In the Caribbean, however, the British were not so fortunate and were blocked by the Spanish in their search for medicinal plants, including Aloe *vera*.

As a result of their shortage of a natural Aloe source, it was the traders in the Cape who sold Aloe juice to the Dutch East India Company, who then exported it to Britain. In the first year of commercial production in 1761, over 90 kg (200 lb) of Aloe sap were sent to Britain. Unfortunately, South African Aloe was not considered as good as the Aloe from Barbados and Socotra. Its main use in South Africa was for rubbing into sprains, and easing rheumatic pain and sciatica. By contrast, in Europe it was used traditionally for the skin and as a digestive aid for the stomach.

The therapeutic and commercial worth of Aloe *ferox* is noted by Sir Joseph Hooker in the *London Journal of Botany* (1842–4). Hooker received his information from Charles Bunbury, FLS, who had accompanied the Governor of the Cape, Sir George Napier, on a journey from Cape Town through to Grahamstown, Fort Beaufort and back to Cape Town. Bunbury mentions that

'Aloe *ferox* is the most important medicine plant of the Colony' and that 'exports of Aloes in one year amounted to £2,794'.[7]

As the commercial value of Aloe was being realized by merchants and traders, so there was added interest in the plant by the great collectors and botanists of Europe. These were frequently aristocratic or rich families who could indulge their collecting passion. Among these number the Prince of Salm-Dyck (1773–1861), who kept the finest collection of succulent plants in Europe, including Aloes. He also wrote a monograph of the Aloe family which appeared in seven parts. In Britain, many landed families had their own greenhouses and exotic plant collections. Both the Dukes of Devonshire and Bedford had especially fine collections.

In Britain, the first modern significant document regarding the medicinal uses of Aloe *vera* was written at the turn of the 20th century by Sir George Watt, a British physician. He lists 43 different medical uses for Aloe *vera* in *A Dictionary of the Economic Products of India* (1908). Sir George was serving with British troops in India at the time, and no doubt drew on Ayurvedic sources for the use of Aloe. He documents some of the following uses:

- fresh juice of Aloe, mixed with milk and water, as a remedy for gonorrhea and methritis
- treatment for melancholia, brain diseases and haemorrhoids
- mixed with alcohol for hair growth (as both Pliny and Dioscorides had noted 18 centuries earlier)
- in infants it was also used (with gum asafoetida) to treat pneumonia and as a paste for the treatment of pleurisy

- rubbed with opium, myrrh and white of egg into swellings, to 'soothe and relieve pain'.[8]

Aloe was also used to treat diseases of the spleen, and to cure intestinal worms in children, treat eye, ear or nose infections. Used to make a sweetmeat, halwa, it was used for piles with 'good effect'. It was also used in veterinary medicine.

The Flora of South Africa by Dr R Marloth, published between 1931 and 1932, has a brief account of some Aloe species. Subsequently an Aloe was named after Marloth, called Aloe *marlothii*, a very distinctive tall-stemmed species found growing in abundance in the Transvaal, northern Natal, Swaziland and Zululand. In 1908, the genus was monographed by Alwin Berger in Engler's *Das Pflanzenreich*. Alwin Berger was the Curator for many years of the gardens of Sir Thomas and Lady Hanbury at 'La Mortala' near Ventimiglia in Italy. This famous garden consisted of 100 acres and 5,000 species. It was rich in Aloes, a great deal of which had been raised from seed and many of which had come from South Africa. Although Berger never visited South Africa and never saw Aloe in its natural habitat, his work is considered remarkably accurate.

Dr I B Pole Evans, CMG, has also been eminent for his contributions to the botanical history of South Africa and for his particular interest in the Aloe family. He was Director of the Botanical Survey of the Union of South Africa as well as being Chief of the Division of Plant Industry, Department of Agriculture in Pretoria during the 1930s. It was in Pretoria that he brought together a very fine collection of Aloes and other plants. He is commemorated in the Aloe *pole-evansii*, a distinctive species collected near Kisumu in Kenya. A major quarterly,

The Flowering Plants of South Africa owed its first 19 volumes to his Pole Evans' editorship. In this work the Aloes of southern and tropical Africa have been systematically represented, with descriptions of no fewer than 100 of the Aloe species.

Modern Times:
Aloe Vera's Medical Uses

PART TWO

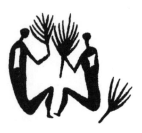

20th-Century Advances

For centuries, Aloe *vera* has been widely used as an effective healing plant, its influence pervading many countries and cultures. Its reputation does not, however, lie only in the romantic realm of folklore and popular mythology. Following on from the work of Pliny, Galen and others, the medical and curative uses of Aloe *vera* were documented in various European journals between the 2nd and 17th centuries. Its chemical analysis, however, only effectively began in the mid-19th century.

It was then known as 'aloin', a bitter brown or black substance extracted from Aloes. This was the only chemical extract that had been broken down and identified. Even today, 'aloin' is still Aloe *vera*'s only recognized active ingredient, and the extract by which it is referred to in established medical circles. In the original *United States Pharmacopoeia* (1922) it is listed under the category Aloes (Bitter Aloes). In the *British Pharmaceutical Codex* of 1907, the extracts aloin and emodin are identified, and Aloe's main value is said to lay in its use as a purgative. It was rarely prescribed on its own, and thus in powdered form as an extract Aloe became one of the most common domestic medicines used as the basis for the majority of patented pills.

Only in the 1930s did serious work begin on the study of Aloe *vera*, in an effort to examine its uses and establish its credibility in contemporary Western medicine. The two chief countries where research has been carried out are the US and Russia, although considerable work has also been carried out in Japan.

Early US Case Histories

In the US, the first work on Aloe *vera* to arouse scientific interest was that of father-and-son team Dr C E Collins and Dr Creston Collins from Maryland in 1935, who treated roentgen (or X-ray) dermatitis with the whole leaf of Aloe *vera*. A woman with a patch of severe roentgen dermatitis on her forehead had received various treatments without success – in fact, her condition worsened. Doctors were about to apply a skin graft but, as a temporary measure, gave her fresh whole Aloe *vera* leaves to reduce her extreme itching and discomfort (doctors based this decision on their knowledge of the use of Aloe *vera* on severe sunburn). Collins and Collins split the leaf to remove the rind and macerated the gel inside, which was applied directly to the woman's skin, covered with wax paper and bound in place with a bandage. Within 24 hours the itching and burning sensation had 'entirely subsided' and, within five weeks, 'there was complete regeneration of the skin of the forehead and scalp, new hair growth, complete restoration of sensation and absence of scar.'[1] Five months after the treatment was started, this woman was completely cured.

From 1934 to 1935, Collins and Collins treated more than 50 cases of X-ray and radium burns with Aloe *vera* leaf and an ointment named 'Alvagel', made from the leaf. X-ray treatment at that time was somewhat crude and often caused burns to the patient. Fresh Aloe *vera* leaves could be wrapped on the wounds every two hours, with no side-effects. In 1935 Dr Creston Collins reported that while 'they have not been perfect cures, the results as a whole have been most gratifying.'[2]

In 1936 Dr C S Wright treated eight cases of radiation telangiectasis (abnormal enlargement of blood vessels), but the only benefit was an improvement in skin texture. With two cases of long-standing X-ray ulceration, however, the results were good. One doctor's hand was almost completely healed from accidental acute radiation dermatitis three weeks after starting the Aloe *vera* treatment.

These and other reports aroused interests in dermatologists and, in 1937, Dr J E Crewe reported on a wider application of Aloe *vera*. Not only was it used with some success to treat eczema, but it had also yielded positive signs for treating ulcers on amputation stumps.

The demand for the fresh leaves of Aloe *vera* grew so great that doctors had difficulty getting hold of them. The Missouri Botanical Garden supplied leaves for fresh radiation burns, but could not provide an inexhaustible supply. Some medical practitioners started propagating their own Aloe *vera* plants to ensure availability and low cost.

In 1938, Dr Archie Fine and Dr Samuel Brown of Cincinnati reported on the successful use of fresh Aloe *vera* leaf in radiology burns. They noted that patients undergoing prolonged radiation therapy, with the consequence that their skin became irritated and painful, experienced considerable soothing of their skin and decreased discomfort with the application of fresh Aloe *vera* leaf. This was particularly noticeable in breast cancer cases, where the armpit became painful after large amounts of radiation. The skin was soothed and pain reduced by the application of Aloe.

In 1939, the treatment of five cases of radiation ulcers, including ulceration in the mouth, with Aloe *vera* gel was reported by Dr Frederick Mandeville, Professor of Radiology at the Medical College of Virginia. The gel healed the mouth ulcers and rapidly relieved the pain. The method used was tedious, however: the patient had to hold the gel in his mouth for about seven hours a day over eight weeks. Although this was troublesome, the condition was serious enough to warrant this effort and proved effective in reducing pain and healing the ulcers.

Most of the literature of the 1930s, therefore, consists of these case histories written by doctors. They were not clinical studies in which double blind controls were used. The authors of these reports, however, were medically trained and familiar with the effects of radiation burns.

Clinical Evidence

The first major attempt to analyse the phyto-chemical constituents of the Aloe *vera* leaf was made by Rowe and others in the early 1940s. In 1940, Professor Tom Rowe of the Medical College in Virginia conducted tests on 25 white rats exposed to high levels of radiation in a laboratory, using Aloe *vera* gel. These initial tests produced variable results, but Professor Rowe concluded that the 'probability that there is a benefit with the jell is 9/10. This is not considered certainty.'[3] He also concluded that too few animals had received treatment, and the period for treatment of two weeks was too short.

In 1941, a second set of experiments using 44 rats was also inconclusive. The results showed that 64 per cent of the rats with radiation burns, treated with Aloe *vera* gel, showed an increased rate of healing. What was more interesting was that different shipments of leaves gave different results. Fresh rind from one shipment gave 100 per cent complete healing within six days for eight rats. Rind from two other shipments gave negative results. The researchers concluded that 'the healing agent of the leaf is concentrated in the rind.'[4] The condition of the leaves and times of collection were also thought to be variable factors in their healing efficacy. Significantly, the researchers also concluded that the 'pulp does not have to be fresh in order to be effective as a healing agent'.[5]

In 1949, the Michigan Department of Health conducted a study on anti-bacterial substances in seed plants. It was subsequently discovered that two aloes contained anti-bacterial agents. These were Aloe *chinensis* and Aloe *succotrina* (regional names for Aloe *vera*). The researchers concluded that there is an 'anti-bacterial principal in Aloe *vera* which inhibits the growth of tubercule bacillii ... found to be the glycoside barbaloin.'[6]

In 1959 in the US, Aloe *vera* finally gained some degree of medical respectability when the FDA (US Food and Drug Administration) reported that '... upon review, the FDA admits that the [Aloe] ointment does actually regenerate skin tissue.'[7] Aloe *vera* was indeed not only highly effective in healing radiation burns but also actively contributes to the regeneration of tissue. Burn patients, in most cases, recovered without scarring.

In 1978, progress was made following Rowe's inconclusive attempt in 1941 to analyse the constituents of Aloe *vera* by Waller and others from the Department of Biochemistry, Oklahoma State University. They confirmed that Aloe *vera* contained 17 amino acids, anti-inflammatory fatty acids, free monosaccharides and polysaccharides, sterols and triterpenoids. A comprehensive survey of the chemical constituents found in Aloe *vera* can be found in Part Four.

Russian Studies

Meanwhile, in Russia in the 1950s, attention was also being directed to the uses of Aloe in radiological departments. In 1956–7 a study by Rostoski and Nordvinov of the Ministry of Health and Chemical Department of the All-Union Research Institute of Medicinal and Aromatic Plants reported on the use of Aloe emulsion in radiation injuries. It was found to be 'one of the most effective preparations when tested on radiation therapy of 200 patients with various ... malignant tumours'.[8]

In this case the Aloe species was almost certainly either Aloe *arborescens* or Aloe *striatula*, which works in the same way as Aloe *vera* but grows more easily in Russia. Medical practitioners found it useful in gynaecology, in the treatment of a skin disease of the vulva characterized by dryness and itching, chiefly affecting older women and often leading to cancer. Aloe emulsion was also used for minor disorders such as cuts, blisters, frostbite and sunburn. The researchers concluded that Aloe reduced the sensitivity of the skin to irradiation and accelerated the healing process, reducing the time for healing from 30–45 days to 15–16 days.

In the same period, 1956–7, S Levenson and K Somova from the Irkukak Medical Institute studied the use of Aloe extract for the treatment of periodontitis, a gum disease. More than 150 patients were treated with oral injections of Aloe mixed with procaine hydrochloride. The course of treatment included 30 injections, with a break for five days half-way through the treatment. Levenson and Somova noted that after 12–15 injections the patients 'indicate a sensation of freshness in the oral cavity and a feeling of stability of the teeth'. At the end of the course, the gum resumed its normal colour and any swelling disappeared.[9]

One Russian study discovered the presence of salicylic acid and cinnamonic acid in Aloe *vera*. Both substances are known anti-microbial agents. In addition, salicylic acid acts as a pain-killer while cinnamonic acid is an anthelmintic – that is, an agent which destroys or prevents infections caused by parasitic worms. The Russian discovery of the presence of traumatic acid in Aloe *vera* sap or rind was used with highly successful results in ulcer treatment. Traumatic acid is a 'wound hormone' of plants and is found in the outer rind or skin of many plants. Thirty years later, in 1982, the presence of salicylic acid in Aloe *vera* was confirmed in findings by the University of Chicago Burn Center. These findings also confirmed that this aspirin-like compound is a breakdown product from aloin (barbaloin), found in the sap of the Aloe *vera* plant.

Dentistry and Veterinary Trials

In 1966 a Dr Bovik, a qualified dentist, reported on the use of Aloe *vera* gel in various dental conditions. In 1970 further reports were made on the use of Aloe *vera* gel to reduce pain and accelerate healing after periodontal surgery. Reduced pain and swelling was observed with the use of Aloe *vera* gel. Russian dental research had already shown that Aloe successfully treats diseases of the bone.

In the 1980s the most extensive study on Aloe *vera*'s use in dentistry was carried out by Dr Bill Wolfe in conjunction with Dr Eugene Zimmerman and the Baylor College of Dentistry, Dallas, Texas. Dr Wolfe concluded that Aloe *vera* was virucidal, bactericidal and fungicidal. Aloe *vera* gel should be applied to the affected area in the mouth as often as possible, either with cotton wool or the fingers. Zimmerman concluded that the bactericidal effects of Aloe *vera* were only evident when a 70 per cent concentration was used. Aloe *vera* had anti-inflammatory qualities without any of the toxic side-effects that other drugs exhibited. It was effective not only for sore areas in the mouth but could also be used under dentures or rubbed around permanent crowns.

In 1975 the use of Aloe *vera* gel in veterinary medicine was described by Northway, who treated a number of external conditions in 76 animals (including 42 dogs, 22 cats and 4 horses) over a period of 1 to 4 weeks, with topical treatment being applied 1 to 4 times a day. His reports ranged from 'good' to 'excellent' in the treatment of various types of inflammation, fungal infections, allergies, abscesses and ringworm. Pain and itching were also relieved after application. Poor results or no changes were noted in only four cases.

In 1980, experiments were undertaken in the use of Aloe *vera* for frostbite in rabbits' ears. Tissue survival was better with the use of Aloe *vera* than without.

In that same year, other researchers reported in detail two cases where commercial Aloe *vera* cream was used to treat severe thermal burns in dogs. This study was followed up with treatment of a Rhesus monkey, accidentally scalded and suffering from 70 per cent burns. After sedation and being put on a drip,

Aloe *vera* cream was applied topically. Within 7 days tissue recovery was extensive; a complete recovery was reported after 30 days.

Note

Further contemporary research on the skin, digestive system, AIDS, cancer, heart disease and other specific illnesses, together with their implications for current medical knowledge, will be dealt with in more detail in the chapters to follow.

Aloe Vera as a Wound-healing Agent

ALOE VERA

It is clear that the bulk of early research on Aloe *vera* has been related to skin disorders, particularly burns and wounds. As a result, it has drawn the attention of dermatologists worldwide in recent years, both for its first-aid applications and for its efficacy in dealing with a wide range of skin complaints.

Bill Coats, a pharmacist and founder of Aloe Vera of America, who has developed a proven stabilization formula for preserving Aloe *vera*, cites the remarkable fact that in southern Texas and northern Mexico, where Aloe *vera* grows abundantly and is used locally, 'there are more than a million people and not one registered dermatologist.'[1] Regular use of Aloe *vera* has meant that 'diseases of the skin, or at least complications arising from them' are minimal.

Burns

Some of the most significant and recent scientific work on burns in the US over the last two decades has been carried out by Dr Heggers (formerly of the University of Chicago Burn Center) and Professor Davis and colleagues.

In 1979, the University of Chicago Burn Center showed that Aloe *vera* seemed to stop progressive injuries due to burns. Research continued, with the result that Aloe *vera* was found to be an effective pain-inhibitor, antibiotic and cell-stimulator. Dr Heggers and his team attributed the ability of Aloe *vera* to heal third-degree burns and frost bite to the salicylates in the plant, and fatty acids such as cholesterol. They reported that Aloe contains anti-inflammatory agents which are less toxic to cell cultures than synthetic anti-inflammatories. Furthermore, the barbaloin in Aloe *vera* makes it highly effective as an anti-microbial agent.

Heggers, therefore, confirmed the findings of previous research done by others such as Gottshall, Brasher and Zimmermann. In 1983, Heggers stated that it was the sap (*anthraquinone glucosides*), and not the gel found within the Aloe *vera* leaves, which was responsible for his results. Ten years on, he wrote:

> Aloe is a product which has a therapeutic potential in a wide variety of devastating soft tissue injuries. Aloe promotes wound healing in the thermal injury ... collective combined data substantiates that Aloe is as recorded in ancient manuscripts a drug of enormous therapeutic potential. It penetrates injured tissue, relieves pain, it is anti-inflammatory and dilates capillaries and increases the blood supply to the injured area ...[2]

Cuts and Wounds

Aloe *vera* is a well-known anti-inflammatory and wound-healer, accelerating the rapid growth of epithelial tissue. According to British dermatologist Dr Peter Atherton, the epithelium is 'an anatomical term which is defined as a layer of cells lining the surface of the body, or a cavity that communicates with it'.[3] Aloe is very effective in healing the range of open wounds or infections like cuts, wounds, boils and abscesses. Aloe *vera* gel or ointment draws out any infection; the flesh cleans itself and facilitates rapid healing. Remarkably, the use of Aloe *vera* in healing wounds can facilitate healing by more than 50 per cent.

Aloin, which is the exudate of Aloe, has direct anti-microbial qualities. This was tested in 1964 by Lorenzetti and others. Leaves were cut, the juice drained out and then the leaves used directly on wounds. This proved effective against *Staphylococcus aureus*, but only when the leaves used were fresh.

Cleaning wounds is part of a cellular process known as 'phagocytosis'.[4] According to biochemist Dr Plaskett, who trains practitioners in Nutritional Medicine and publishes scientific research on Aloe *vera* under the auspices of the Aloe Vera Information Service, based in Cornwall, England, in this process 'the immune system mops up and banish[es] from the body, bacteria and other infective agents, and other debris, such as arises when tissue cells die.'[5]

Aloe *vera* contains a growth-promoting factor which enhances the healing process in wounds. An address to the 6th International Congress on Traditional and Folk Medicine in December 1992 in Texas by Dr Heggers and others confirmed that Aloe, used topically, is very effective in wound-healing. Wounds treated only with Aloe *vera* healed faster than those treated by any other means.

From 1987 onwards, far-reaching studies have been carried out specifically in relation to wound-healing by Professor Robert H Davis and others. They have examined evidence that Aloe *vera* is effective in treating wounds and reducing inflammation by the action of one of Aloe's major sugars, mannose-6 phosphate. They concluded that mannose-6 phosphate 'is an important factor in the wound healing process and plays a significant role in the biological activity of Aloe *vera*'.[6]

Another study by Professor Davis and his colleagues suggests that Aloe's 'watery composition may increase the migration of epithelial cells so that an improvement of wound healing is recorded ... epithelial cells proliferate ... and eventually cover the wound with skin'.[7] They also observed that 'animals not receiving topical Aloe had hard and crusty wounds, which generally appeared unclean. However, the Aloe-treated wounds were clean, with healthy granulation tissue.'[8] They concluded that Aloe could possibly improve wound-healing by increasing oxygen availability and collagen strength. It is effective orally, which suggests it is taken directly into the bloodstream (and not broken down by the digestive tract). Aloe *vera* can topically reduce inflammation. It has been called a 'biogenic stimulator' or a 'wound hormone' by the German pharmacist, Freytag.

In 1994, Professor Davis and others claimed that 'gibberellin, isolated from Aloe, increased wound-healing more than 100 per cent in mice.'[9] Little other work appears to have been done on gibberellin except in a paper by Davis on Aloe *vera* and its effect on wound-healing in people with diabetes. This paper reports on diabetic ulcers affecting the lower extremities of the body. For someone with diabetes, an ulcer can prove life-threatening. In the US each year, 14 per cent of patients with diabetes require hospitalization for foot problems. Aloe *vera* contains ingredients such as vitamin E, zinc and ascorbic acid, all powerful wound-healers. It is also anti-inflammatory and anti-oedemic – that is, it reduces swelling. Davis and his colleagues noted that 'the diabetic patient suffers from a diminished wound healing mechanism, an insensitivity to pain perception, and altered fluid dynamics, resulting in a prolonged edema response.'[10]

Tests were done on mice to verify these properties. The conclusions were remarkable: 'As an aid in promotion diabetic wound healing, test groups treated with A. *vera* displayed nearly a 100 per cent increase in wound size reduction as compared to their untreated counterparts.'[11] Mice treated with Aloe *vera* had three times the tolerance to pain of untreated mice. In terms of swelling, the animals treated with Aloe *vera* showed a five-fold reduction in swelling compared to the untreated diabetic mice.

Scars

Aloe *vera* is known to have a marked effect in the treatment of scar tissue. It is also effective in helping to prevent scarring, following injury to the skin. This is because Aloe *vera* stimulates cell production through the activity of the amino acids, which are the basis for new cell formation, and because its enzymes promote regeneration at the deepest layers of the skin.

Research into the effects of Aloe *vera* on scar tissue has been carried out in the field of dermabrasion, which aims to remove scars in acne patients. This radical process literally shaves away the epidermis and scar tissue with high-speed brushes to allow the skin to reconstitute itself. This is a risky and painful process and generally healing is slow. If unsuccessful, it can lead to greater disfigurement. It is more commonly used in the US than in Britain.

Dr Peter Atherton became interested in Aloe *vera* after reading a paper published by the Acne Research Institute of California documenting the use of Aloe *vera* gel in post-dermabrasion wound-healing. In this experiment Aloe *vera* gel was added to the post-operative dressing on only one side of the face. The other side of the face was given the normal post-operative dressing. The side which had the Aloe *vera* gel increased the rate of healing by 25–30 per cent.

Ulcers

Aloe *vera* can be used successfully in the general treatment of skin ulcers ranging from mouth ulcers to cold sores (herpes simplex), genital ulcers and serious leg ulcers.

Cold sores or fever blisters (two somewhat contradictory popular names for herpes simplex) affect countless people, generally around the mouth or other moist areas of the body such as the eyes, ears or nose. Herpes simplex in the eyes can cause blindness. Aloe *vera* gel, being anti-virucidal, is effective in curing herpes simplex over a period of up to three days. It is even more effective in treating herpes zoster, otherwise known as shingles.

Research carried out in the 1970s stated that 'Aloe *vera* is bactericidal to at least [six] species of bacteria, especially to the more common strept and staph infections ... In an 80 per cent concentration, it is broadly virucidal ... It is virucidal to four members of the Herpes virus strain including Herpes simplex and Herpes zoster. In an 80 per cent concentration, it is fungicidal against yeast infections ...'[12]

Bill Coats documents the extraordinary story of a woman suffering from herpes simplex in the eyes, who lost her sight in her left eye for five days, and then, when she'd recovered, in her right eye for six weeks. She used Aloe *vera* gel three times daily, squirting it directly into the severely infected right eye. This allowed her to see within a few days. At the same time she was drinking Aloe *vera* juice. After eight weeks not only had the infection cleared up but most of the scarring that accompanies herpes simplex had disappeared.

In 1987, Dr Rosalie Burns MD, a professor and chairman of the Department of Neurology at The Medical College of Pennsylvania, reported on the effect of Aloe *vera* on shingles (Herpes zoster). Common herpes of the mouth and sexual organs, as well as chicken pox, are caused by the same virus that causes shingles. Once a child recovers from chicken pox, the virus lies dormant in the spinal nerves in the body, mostly inactive. When it is reactivated, however, it appears as shingles. Dr Burns concluded that: 'Sap from the leaves of the Aloe *vera* plant is an old folk remedy that relieves pain and speeds healing when spread over the blisters.'[13]

In 1973 two Egyptian doctors, Dr El Zawahry, MD, Professor of Dermatology at Cairo University and Dr Hegazy, MD, produced a paper on the use of Aloe *vera* in treating three sufferers with chronic leg ulcers and dermatoses. Generally chronic leg ulcers are difficult to treat as they are resistant to treatment.

Fresh Aloe *vera* gel was used, homogenized and refrigerated with the addition of a preservative. This was used for one month. The gel was applied topically on the ulcers three to five times a day after the lesions had been cleaned. Occasionally antibiotics and antihistamines were also given (considering that Aloe *vera* has both antibiotic and antihistaminic properties, this was perhaps slightly over-cautious).

The first case was of a man with two ulcers on his left leg, surrounded by eczema, from which he had suffered for 15 years. One ulcer was large, the other small. Both smelt foul. Within the first week of treatment tissue healing was noted in the larger ulcer, which had not responded to any previous treatment. After four weeks the smaller ulcer showed improvement, and after six weeks had completely healed. After 11 weeks, the lower part of the larger ulcer was completely healed, while the upper part remained but had shrunk in size. The other two cases showed similarly satisfactory results.

Zawahry and his colleagues believed that the active ingredient in the healing was the mucopolysaccharides. Their conclusions: 'Aloe *vera* proved to have a stimulating effect on the rate of healing of chronic leg ulcers ...'[14]

It should be noted that these were case studies and not clinical trials.

Skin and Hair Care

Over the last 20 years, interest in the beautifying properties of Aloe *vera* has risen dramatically. This is reflected in the number of cosmetic products and toiletries which are available today that include Aloe *vera* amongst their main active ingredients. Major cosmetics firms have incorporated it into their products to take advantage of the age-old reputation of Aloe *vera* as a skin-healer, skin softener, moisturizer and anti-ageing agent.

It is commonly believed that the moisturizing, emollient and healing properties of Aloe gel are due to the polysaccharides present: the major polysaccharide present being *glucomannan*. According to Dr Albert Leun, however, it is probable that 'the gel's beneficial properties are not due to the polysaccharides alone but rather from a synergistic effect of these compounds with other substances present in the gel.'[1]

Dermatologist Dr Peter Atherton has enthusiastically taken up the use of Aloe *vera* in his own practice. He has tested its efficacy amongst a selected group of patients. The two areas in which he considers Aloe *vera* most effective is as a skin treatment and for boosting the immune system.

Dr Atherton lists the four main cosmetic properties of Aloe *vera* as follows:

1 it acts as a moisturizer

2 it increases collagen

3 it reduces pigment formation

4 it enhances the skin's immune system.

Research Findings

- Aloe *vera* has the ability to moisturize through the action of its polysaccharides. These help to provide the skin with water-binding abilities, thereby restoring and retaining moisture.

- Aloe *vera* feeds the skin with a wide range of vitamins, minerals and nutrients.

- Aloe *vera* gel increases the creation of collagen production, the skin's support protein, through increasing human fibroblast cells six to eight times faster than normal cell production. Fibroblast cells produce the fibres of scar tissue to knit wounds; the more there are, the more rapid will be the healing.

- Aloe *vera* stimulates cell production through the activity of amino acids. It is rich in amino acids, which are the basis for new cell formation. Aloe *vera* provides 20 out of the 22 amino acids the body needs for growth.

- Aloe *vera* stimulates cell production without the risk of cancer, as it is non-toxic.

- Aloe *vera* reduces and eliminates brown spots or age spots through its anti-tyrosinase activity.

- Aloe *vera* enhances the skin's immune system through its polysaccharides, which allow protection against ultraviolet rays.

- Use of Aloe *vera* provides a natural pH protection as it has almost the same pH factor as skin. It simultaneously cleanses the skin, removes bacteria and supplies nourishment.

- Aloe *vera* has a tightening, astringent action which reduces large pores and thereby the possibility of blemishes. This takes place through the action of the polysaccharides, which have, according to research, the ability to reorganize the skin's epidermal cells in the upper layer of the skin. With age these cells become looser, moisture escapes more readily and bacteria have readier access to the skin. As the epidermal cells tighten through the use of Aloe *vera*, moisture levels rise, skin looks younger and a protective barrier against the pollution of the modern world is restored.

- The polysaccharides also create a barrier which prevents moisture loss.

- Combined with lignin, also found in Aloe *vera* gel, the polysaccharides help Aloe *vera* to penetrate through seven layers of the skin, allowing deep absorption. Aloe can then be used with other ingredients such as vitamin E or Spirulina to enhance skin beauty, its penetrating action allowing other ingredients to enter right into the skin's inner layers. Combined with Aloe *vera* gel, water can also be taken deep down through seven layers of skin. This is one of its most potent qualities in the possibility of creating and retaining youthful skin.

- Aloe *vera*, by promoting blood circulation, restores a healthy colour to the skin.
- The enzymes in Aloe *vera* slough off dead cells so that new tissue can form. This allows the pores to breathe, throws off older tougher skin and makes the skin more youthful looking. This enzymatic activity can reduce or eliminate scars, age lines and blemishes.
- Aloe *vera* detoxifies the skin through the presence of uronic acids.
- Aloe *vera*'s anti-inflammatory activity prohibits the growth of bacteria, including *staphylococcus*.
- Aloe *vera* works on greasy skin by mopping up excess oil, thus preventing acne or clearing it up. At the same time, Aloe *vera* is a good moisturizer when combined with water (in the case of very dry skin, however, Aloe *vera* should be combined with a good moisturizing agent).
- Aloe *vera* has naturally anti-allergenic properties and is also naturally antibiotic. It can therefore be used on sensitive skin.

Acne

Acne responds very well to topical treatment of Aloe *vera*. Doctor and dermatologist Lawrence Meyerson of Texas has reported excellent results treating a more severe form of acne which causes scarring, known as acne *vulgaris*, with Aloe *vera* gel. One hundred cases were treated with excellent results, resulting in relief 'of pain and itching, subsiding of infection' and reduction of scar tissue. There was no noted toxicity.[2]

In 1973 Dr Zawahry and his colleagues in Egypt treated three women between 18 and 25 years old with mixed acne *vulgaris*. Aloe *vera* treatment lasted one month. At the end of this, two of the patients were completely free from acne lesions, while the third showed a 'marked improvement with minimal residual acne lesions'.[3]

Ageing Skin

The skin covers the entire body and reflects the ageing process with uncanny accuracy. Aloe *vera* has been shown to slow down the ageing process through several actions: it is an excellent cleanser, sloughing off old cells and cleaning the pores. It has a detoxifying effect on the skin by removing wastes and toxins, and its vitamins, minerals and amino acids nourish the skin. Amino acids also stimulate new cell growth.

Studies have shown that Aloe *vera*'s legendary anti-ageing properties lie in the plant's amazing capacity to produce fibroblast cells six to eight times faster than normal cells. These cells manufacture collagen, which keeps skin firm. Hands will become softer and smoother as Aloe allows the skin to rejuvenate itself at a cellular level. Aloe's keratolytic action also breaks down and softens hard skin on the feet and hands, restoring its suppleness.

Retin-A, known in the medical world as retinoic acid, has enjoyed popularity as a prescription drug with anti-ageing qualities. It has the same action as the polysaccharides in Aloe *vera*, making the epidermal cells fit more tightly together. This cell density reduces wrinkles but unfortunately has side-effects such as skin irritation. Aloe *vera* does not irritate the skin like Retin-A.

Allergies and Itching

Aloe *vera* acts as an anti-allergenic for 99 per cent of the population. A pain inhibitor due to the presence of salicylic acid (found in aspirin) and bradykinose, it may prove to be an even more potent source of pain relief since it also alleviates itching. Russian research has shown that Aloe *vera* enables the body to deal with harmful substances, and so it can be useful when there are negative allergic reactions to other substances.

One woman of 64 years had a severe case of pruritis – the skin of her vulva was thickened and the inner part of her thighs were thick and purplish – relieved by Aloe *vera*. Previous treatments had not alleviated her itching and burning and she had become highly nervous and unable to sleep without the help of sedatives. Aloe ointment was applied with almost immediate relief in terms of the itching, burning sensation. Within two weeks the skin had become normal, swelling had reduced and there was no irritation.

Eczema

Barcroft cites a case history of a child with eczema, treated by an alternative practitioner. The girl was four years old and almost entirely covered with eczema, causing her to scratch her skin through constant irritation. She was bathed daily in spring water with Dead Sea salt added. Afterwards Aloe *vera* juice was applied directly onto the eczematous skin. It was also taken orally in small doses throughout the day, along with some blue-green algae. Her diet was adjusted to cut down on dairy products, white flour and white sugar. Initially the eczema worsened, but slowly over six months the severity lessened until it was 90 per cent better!

Hair Care (Hair Loss and Dandruff)

Aloe *vera* benefits the hair and scalp in much the same way as it benefits our skin. Hair is primarily composed of keratin, which contains mostly amino acids as well as oxygen, carbon and traces of hydrogen, sulphur and nitrogen. Laurie Taylor-Donald claims that Aloe *vera* has a chemical composition very similar to keratin and this helps revitalize the hair with nutrients. The growth of healthy hair, then, depends on a healthy scalp which is supplied by blood vessels feeding into the hair papilla – a small elevation at the end of the root. If the skin is affected, the hair will also suffer.

Dandruff (*seborrhea sicca*) and baldness (*alopecia*) are the two most common disorders affecting the hair and scalp. *Seborrhea* arises from excessive oil in the skin. *Seborrhea sicca* is characterized by itching and small white scales in the hair and/or on the scalp. *Seborrhea oleosa* is greasy dandruff: sebum mixes with the scaly scalp, causing stickiness. If these greasy scales come off, bleeding or oozing may result and medical attention should be sought. It is an altogether more serious condition than the dry dandruff condition.

Hair falling out in patches is known as *alopecia areata*. This can be triggered by sudden shock, illness or injury. If the nervous system is traumatized in any way, the blood flow to the scalp is affected. If the effects of trauma continue to affect blood flow over a prolonged period, the hair follicles become deprived of blood and this causes hair to fall out.

Scalp conditions can also cause ill health in the hair such as eczema or psoriasis. Aloe *vera* has showed itself successful in treating both eczema and psoriasis and research has also been done on the use of Aloe *vera* in treating hair and scalp conditions.

Research Findings

- Aloe *vera* is both fungicidal and bactericidal. Dandruff and *seborrhea* are fungal infections formed in a base of sebum.

- The enzymes in Aloe *vera* cast off dead cells to allow new tissue to form.

- The amino acids present in Aloe *vera* facilitate the growth of healthy tissue. The amino acids complex in Aloe *vera* is the same complex functioning in healthy papilla and hair follicles.

- The deep penetrating action of the polysaccharides and lignin in Aloe *vera* brings deep cleansing to the scalp and allows nutrients to penetrate.

- The same deeply penetrating action allows Aloe *vera* to work below the scalp surface as an anti-infectious agent at the same time as it revitalizes dead tissue.

- Aloe *vera* is anti-pruritic and soothes scalp itching.

- The saponins in Aloe *vera* are natural cleansing and soap-producing agents which both clean and strengthen the hair.

- Aloe *vera*, combined with jojoba, provides a shampoo which can combat *seborrhea* and other conditions as well as restore the hair to shining health.

Research is being undertaken in the US to see whether Aloe *vera* can stimulate new growth if hair roots are not dead. There is already some clinical evidence that suggests this is possible.

Psoriasis

Although it is considered that there is no actual cure for psoriasis, it can be contained and largely healed with Aloe *vera*. As psoriasis is linked to the general nutritional well-being of the skin, Aloe *vera* should be taken internally as well as used topically on the inflamed area. In 1975 Bill Coats documented more than 25 cases of psoriasis treated successfully in one year with Aloe *vera*, megavitamins and a strict diet which excluded convenience foods, sugars and excessive animal fat. One young man's condition cleared up almost completely after 90 days of treatment.

Some of the most important work to appear recently was that presented at the Fourth Congress of The European Academy of Dermatology and Venereology in October 1995: researchers reported that:

> Aloe *vera* extract is a grease-free penetrant which is readily absorbed into dermal and deeper tissues. It carries analgesic, antiallergic, antipruritic, wound-healing and anti-inflammatory components such as amino acids ... [Aloe *vera* kept the skin moist and inhibited] the psoriatic plaques by suppressing proliferation and stimulatory differentiation of the cells in the epidermis.[4]

Anti-inflammatory Properties

ALOE VERA

Inflammation is the body's natural response to any injury and is the initial part of the healing process. It is a complicated procedure characterized by heat and redness, pain and swelling. Some of the medical conditions in which Aloe *vera* is effective as an anti-inflammatory, such as wounds, burns and skin problems, have been dealt with in earlier chapters. All of these involve damage or breakage of the skin.

Aloe *vera*'s anti-inflammatory action has been well researched and is accepted as one of its most fundamental healing actions. There are two processes involved:

> 1 reduction of the inflammation and pain alleviation
> 2 healing of the injury.

This covers not only external injuries such as burns or wounds but internal illnesses which have pronounced inflammatory components. Scientific research confirms that Aloe *vera* is significant in the inhibition of acute inflammation. Work by Professor Davis and others is notable in this regard.

> Aloe *vera* may be the most powerful, non toxic, plant-derived treatment of both inflammation and wound healing. Presently, hydrocortisone

is a most effective treatment for inflammation ... However, while inhibiting inflammation, hydrocortisone blocks wound healing.[1]

Aloe *vera* is one of the few known substances which simultaneously decreases inflammation and promotes healing. Professor Davis tested whether Aloe *vera* and hydrocortisone could be used at the same time. One of the aims of this study was to examine whether Aloe *vera* would be shown to 'mask or negate hydrocortisone's antiwound healing properties'. Research attempted to locate those specific components, out of more than 200 different biological agents, in Aloe *vera* which are both anti-inflammatory and wound-healing.

Steroid drugs exert an anti-inflammatory effect and, since Aloe *vera* contains natural plant sterols, the theory was that Aloe *vera* could act in a similar way to steroid drugs but without their side-effects. Since steroids have undesirable side-effects and are naturopathically suppressive, unlike Aloe, this could be a very significant function of Aloe *vera*.

The principal plant sterols in Aloe *vera* are Lupeol, B-Sisosterol and Campesterol, which were indeed confirmed by this research to be powerful anti-inflammatory agents. The most effective is Lupeol, which had the greatest influence on inflammation reduction (37 per cent). Davis and his researchers concluded that the dose-response curve in Lupeol was remarkably similar to that of Aloe *vera*.

Therefore, Aloe's sterols were definitely responsible, to some extent, for its anti-inflammatory properties. They are not the only properties, however, and it is known that the entire Aloe *vera* plant exhibits bradykininase activity: bradykininase breaks down bradykinin, which stimulates inflammation. Two Japanese studies have shown the presence of the bradykininase enzyme in other healing Aloes, including Aloe *saponaria* and Aloe *arborescens var. natalensis*.

Davis concluded that:

> [The] study does not suggest the use of *A. vera* as a replacement, but rather as an aid for current steroid therapies. It has been the authors' purpose to increase the effectiveness of steroid therapy in the management of inflammation, using a natural substance.[2]

Another factor which may influence inflammation reduction is the presence in Aloe *vera* of salicylic acid. Salicylic acid, which is a close relation of aspirin, has pain-reducing qualities (as does bradykininase) and inhibits the production of certain prostaglandin hormones: hormone-like body chemicals which encourage inflammation. Salicylates are found in fruits such as raspberries, currants, dates, cherries, apples, grapes and prunes, and are also found in wine! Although it is not yet known to what degree Aloe *vera* contains sufficient concentrations of salicylic acid to make this an effective anti-inflammatory, research suggests that salicylic acid has a role to play in Aloe's overall anti-inflammatory action.

There has also been a suggestion that Aloe *vera* has an antihistamine effect. It is uncertain whether this is due to the magnesium in Aloe *vera* or not. What is known is that Aloe *vera* is superb for healing the lining of the bowel, which means that there are fewer food allergy reactions due to 'leaky gut' syndrome.

Angina and Heart Disease

In Britain heart disease is one of the biggest killers, with 150,000 deaths per annum. Significantly, though, according to *The Times* a healthier diet and lifestyle changes, especially among the middle classes, has seen a dramatic reduction of heart disease as a major factor in mortality. Unfortunately, nutritional changes are linked to income and education, and it is still a major disease amongst those who do not or who cannot afford to eat more fruit and vegetables.

Clinical work in relation to Aloe *vera* and heart disease is severely limited. Dr Danhof has found that Aloe *vera* can help to prevent heart attacks in those people who suffer from heart problems or who are predisposed to heart disease through their family history. He recommends taking Aloe *vera* juice daily. This has been confirmed by the one serious and extensive study done on heart disease, which was carried out in India by Dr O P Agarwal. His research findings came to the conclusion that:

> [When Aloe *vera*, mixed with the Husk of Isabgol] was given to the patients of atherosclerotic heart disease, there was a definite and substantial improvement (about 95 per cent) in their clinical profile apart from bio-chemical changes and ECG tracings. These two substances need further evaluation to find out the exact mechanism of action on atherosclerosis.[3]

Alasdair Barcroft refers to studies in which it has been shown that Aloe *vera*-

juice, taken daily, can lower blood pressure within a few weeks and cholesterol levels by 12–14 points.

In 1998 C D Mistry treated the Chief Minister of Bihar, India, who was suffering from 60–70 per cent clogged arteries and angina. He recommended the use of Aloe *vera* with Neem[4] (an oil with stimulative antiseptic and healing properties which has been used successfully for skin problems, ulcers and eczema) together with L. arginine, an amino acid, and high doses of vitamins C and E. Dosage was 30 ml daily of Aloe *vera* and Neem. It took four months before the clogging disappeared. This showed up on an angiograph. After six months the condition was cured. The Minister is still taking Aloe *vera* with Neem to prevent any further clogging of the arteries. He follows a moderate diet excluding cheese, peas, wine and animal fat.

Arthritis

Orthodox medicine usually treats arthritis with anti-inflammatory drugs such as steroids or non-steroidal anti-inflammatories (NSAIDS) such as aspirin and other painkillers. Although these provide relief, ironically the latter treatment is known to encourage gastric ulceration and increase the 'permeability of the intestinal wall'.[5]

With its powerful anti-inflammatory properties, Aloe *vera* has been able to treat arthritis effectively by providing pain relief and joint flexibility. In addition, by increasing the healing and immune potential of the system it can reverse or at least arrest aspects of the disease.

Work has been done on animals with positive results by Professor Davis and colleagues of the Pennsylvania College of Podiatric Medicine in Philadelphia, in

1985 and 1986. In 1985 their work with rats injected with Aloe *vera* (150 mg/kilo) brought about a 72 per cent reduction of arthritic symptoms. Their tests in 1986 showed a positive response again to treating animal arthritis with Aloe *vera*, who specifically responded to the Aloe phenolics, in particular anthraquinone.

Links between arthritis and the digestive system have been made by Dr Jeffrey Bland, formerly at the Linus Pauling Institute of Science and Medicine in California. In 1985 he reported that drinking Aloe *vera* juice showed an improvement in colonic activity and lowered bowel putrefaction. This allowed easier absorption of protein and, according to Dr Bland, may indicate why some individuals have found Aloe *vera* to be helpful in various food allergy symptoms such as arthritic-like pain.

The work of Dr Hemmings shows that incomplete protein breakdown products from foods can be transported via a 'leaky' digestive lining into the bloodstream and initiate either antibody-antigen reactions in the bloodstream, which can aggravate the symptoms of arthritis, or participate in direct antigen assault upon the digestive lining, increasing the risk of inflammatory bowel disorders.

Aloe *vera* can improve the digestive system and protein absorption. When there is poor digestion and poor protein absorption, the antigen-antibody complexes can be trapped in the liver and the joints and initiate inflammatory processes such as pain and swelling. This is why a dietary fast can be helpful in reducing the symptoms of rheumatoid arthritis.

Aloe *vera* is also helpful in the treatment of osteoarthritis. The long-chain mucopolysaccharides in Aloe *vera*, including the most significant component, acemannan, have the ability to enhance or slow down the immune system response. They are found in every cell of the body according to American nutritionist Dr E Harendal. Significantly with regard to arthritis, mucopolysaccharides provide lubrication of the joints; they also line the colon to prevent the absorption of toxic wastes, and facilitate the absorption of water, nutrients and electrolytes in the gastro-intestinal tract.

Asthma

There has been very little available published research in English on the use of Aloe in treating asthma. In Japan three trials were done in the 1980s, and some work has also been done in Russia. This is an area that deserves extensive research, as asthma is such a common problem, particularly in inner cities.

There have been case reports of the successful treatment of asthma through Aloe *vera* by both alternative medical practitioners and as a folk treatment: it has been used in Russia as an inhalant. More importantly, in Russia, Filatow and his colleagues have treated bronchial asthma successfully with Aloe extract in tissue therapy.

Digestion

One of the major ways in which Aloe *vera* is consistently effective is in treating the digestive system. Here its actions are both anti-inflammatory and immune-stimulatory. Not only the gut itself but the entire digestive system has a vast array of immune lymphoid cells throughout its tissues. Their function is vital for digestive health, the health of the intestinal systems, gastric functioning, liver functioning and healthier bowel flora. Individuals suffering from indigestion, colitis, irritable bowel syndrome, Crohn's disease (an inflammatory disease of the small bowel), diverticulitis (this is a condition in which diverticula in the colon are associated with lower abdominal pain), peptic ulcers and excessive stomach acid have all reported relief after taking Aloe *vera* juice. These reports have not been linked to controlled studies but rather to anecdotal evidence. And it should be noted that the treatment of irritable bowel syndrome with Aloe *vera* gel needs to be continuous. If a patient stops taking Aloe *vera*, the symptoms return.[6]

Aloe Vera and the Immune System

The immune system is the body's own protection against foreign invaders such as bacteria and viruses, and destructive elements within the body itself. When it is depleted, illness arises. If we want to maintain our health and capacity to deal with all sorts of infections and viruses, we need to keep our immune system functioning at its optimum level.

A number of factors place our system under stress: increased environmental pollution, a diet depleted of nutritional value, genetically modified food, work and financial insecurity, family and community disintegration, general stress and irregular lifestyles – all these factors contribute to a breakdown of our immune system. More than ever we need to take care to detoxify our bodies and boost our immune system if we are to stay relatively free of disease. Boosting our immune system not only acts as preventative health care but increases our sense of well-being and our capacity for life and enjoyment.

Besides a beneficial diet, exercise and lifestyle, supplements may be necessary to ensure a strong balanced system. Aloe *vera*, with its wide complex of vitamins and minerals and over 200 constituents, is one of the most powerful immuno-stimulants readily available today.

A number of conditions which arise out of a depressed immune system are commonly linked to poor digestive function. Aloe *vera* has been shown to be effective in regulating digestive function.

Aloe *vera* also acts directly on the immune system through one of its principal long-chain sugars (mucopolysaccharides), acemannan. This has been isolated by Dr Bill McAnalley, a pharmacologist at the Carrington Laboratories in the US. Subsequent research on acemannan by Dr McDaniel, a pathologist at the Dallas-Fort Worth Medical Center, has shown in trials with AIDS patients that acemannan is a powerful immuno-stimulant. Acemannan performs the same function as synthetic drugs which are normally used to treat immune-based conditions, but without the side-effects these synthetic treatments can cause.

According to Dr John Pittman, a specialist in immune disorders and Programme Director of the Hippocrates Health Institute in Florida, the acemannan in Aloe *vera* acts directly to enhance the activity of the immune system. It increases the number and intensity of action of the immune cells in the body such as macrophages and the T-cells, as well as the B-cells in the spleen, which form antibodies. Damage to the bone marrow by drugs such as AZT and toxic chemicals is inhibited by the use of acemannan.

Macrophages are white blood cells (part of the immune system) which carry out the process known as 'phagocytosis' which is really a cell 'mopping up' process by which debris linked to toxins and poisons, are digested and destroyed within the body.[1] It is a critical function directly linked to purifying and cleansing the body. Acemannan in Aloe *vera* directly stimulates this action and is therefore an immune system stimulant, without any toxic effects. It has been shown that macrophages, stimulated by acemannan, are 10 times more effective than unstimulated macrophages at killing tumour cells. By stimulating the immune system, it both enhances the body's capacity to fight diseases and enhances healing.

Lectins are also found in plants and have immuno-stimulatory properties. Not all plant lectins are beneficial, but those found in Aloe have been shown to be beneficial as they contain two properties: they activate cells and cause them to divide – a process known as mitosis – and they induce 'cell aggregation and clump formation', known as agglutination.[2]

There are a number of diseases with immune-related components for which Aloe *vera* can have a beneficial effect. These range from AIDS, cancer, ME and Multiple Sclerosis to Type I diabetes, as well as other conditions.

AIDS

In Europe, work was first carried out in Brussels (1988) to research the effect of Aloe *vera* on AIDS. Drs Clumeck and Hermans studied the effect of antiviral drugs on human immunodeficiency virus (HIV). They examined the properties of acemannan, which they called 'carrisyn' and reported that it possessed both anti-viral and immuno-modulating properties. Amongst AIDS patients who took carrisyn, a reduction in infected cells was noted.

The acemannan in Aloe *vera*

has direct effects on the cells of the immune system, activating and stimulating macrophages, monocytes, antibodies and T-cells. [It acts as a bridge between] foreign proteins (such as virus particles) and macrophages, facilitating phagocytosis ... this is a key component in boosting cell-mediated immunity which is deficient in HIV infection. It increases the number and intensity of action of macrophages, killer T-cells, and monocytes, as well as increasing the number of antibody forming B-cells in the spleen. Acemannan also protects the bone marrow from damage by toxic chemicals and drugs such as AZT.[3]

Patients with AIDS treated with Aloe *vera* showed significant improvement, to the extent that some patients were able to return to work. These patients had previously been seriously ill, unable to get out of bed and work or study.[4]

Lee Ritter, who has an almost evangelical enthusiasm towards the use of Aloe *vera*, reports on the remarkable work being done by Dr McDaniel, Chief Pathologist at the Dallas-Fort Worth Medical Center, in Texas. He recounts Dr McDaniel showing him X-rays of an AIDS patient who was given 4 to 21 days to live. He had 17 malignant tumours on his liver, one the size of a cricket ball. With no orthodox medical cure available, this patient started taking Aloe *vera* throughout the day. Six months after taking Aloe *vera* the tumours had completely disappeared. X-rays taken showed only scar tissue.

Dr McDaniel also carried out a pilot study of 16 AIDS patients who were treated with 1,000 mg of acemannan for six months. According to McDaniel, acemannan boosted AIDS patients' immune system without toxic side-effects. After three months patients seriously ill with AIDS showed a 20 per cent improvement; patients less seriously ill showed an improvement of 71 per cent.

Dr David Smallbone cautions that using a specific extract from Aloe *vera* is an acceptable means for research purposes but not necessarily as a therapeutic tool. Isolating acemannan means that other factors, present in Aloe *vera*, that ameliorates its action, may be absent.

Dr Joan Priestley, reputedly one of Los Angeles' leading holistic physicians, is known as the 'AIDS Queen Physician' as she takes care of hundreds of AIDS patients. As part of an integrated AIDS treatment programme which includes nutrition and anti-viral therapy, she recommends high doses of vitamins such as vitamin C and Aloe *vera* extract (AVE) in place of the isolated acemannan or synthetic drugs. Vitamin A, zinc and garlic are also used to boost a failing immune system. Many HIV-positive patients are deficient in minerals and vitamins, and also have a high degree of malabsorption. In her work, Dr Priestley uses the whole-leaf Aloe *vera*, known to be most effective with digestive problems and boosting the immune system. Doses vary between 2 and 8 oz a day depending on the severity of the condition.

Cancer and Tumours

There has been relatively little known scientific research on the effect of Aloe on malignant tumours. Most of the trials on tumours have been done on animals, and have demonstrated Aloe's positive effect on the inhibition of tumour growth. Clinical evidence suggests, therefore, that Aloe *vera* would appear to have a profound anti-cancer effect on the cells.

In Russia early in the 20th century, Aloe was used to treat cancer patients. Extract of Aloe was injected subcutaneously (under the skin). This treatment was combined with a nutritional emphasis on fresh foods, particularly freshly pressed red juices from beets, cherries, blueberries, blackberries, etc. This treatment was helpful in cleansing the system and therefore effective for all diseases of the immune system.[5] As cancers only develop when the immune system is compromised, this approach is only to be commended.

It is interesting to note that the Japanese today are using a vaccination against cancer, known as Maruyama, which works by activating the lymphocytes and boosting the immune system. More than 337,000 people have used Maruyama with strikingly positive results since the early 1970s.[6]

Much of the subsequent work in Japan has employed Aloe *arborescens*, using the whole leaf extract. Again this would include the aloin fraction, which leads to speculation as to its contribution in anti-tumour activity. Research carried out in 1972 by Okada and others showed the successful use of Aloe in inhibiting animal tumours. Subsequent work carried out by the Japanese over the following 21 years has shown that acemannan has both anti-tumour and lectin-like properties. Research on which polysaccharide fractions in Aloe have anti-tumour properties showed that aloctin A, which is an active substance of Aloe *arborescens*, also has an immuno-modulatory action.

In the US, work has been carried out on Aloe extracts used on both normal and tumour cells in vitro. Fractions of leaf extracts from two Aloe varieties, Aloe *vera* and Aloe *saponaria*, were tested for the presence of lectin-like activities and their effect on normal and tumour cells. The conclusions were notable, in that substances in fluid fractions from both leaf sources 'were found to markedly promote attachment and growth of normal human cells, but not tumour cells, and to enhance healing of wounded cell monolayers'. This factor would favour the eventual predominance of normal cells.[7]

One of the most remarkable stories known to the authors is that of C D Mistry BSc, MRPS, ND of Hampstead, London. In 1979 he was diagnosed with a tumour in his lungs and given six months to live. An operation would give him a 50/50 chance. He knew Sir Jason Winter, a gentleman much travelled in the East who had cured himself of a brain tumour with Aloe *vera*. With the odds evenly matched, Mr Mistry decided to embark on a course of Aloe *vera*. After ordering 10 kg of Aloe *vera* juice from America, he started to treat himself. Seriously ill, his belly was very swollen and he had difficulty eating. He was coughing up blood intermittently. After one year the swelling went down and the tumour was not only arrested, it had diminished in size. He continued working hard. This was 20 years ago and Mr Mistry now leads a normal, extremely active life. The tumour is still there but much diminished. According to him, Aloe *vera* 'changed my life'.

Drug Abuse (Recovery Programmes)

A study of the use of Aloe *vera* with drug abusers in the early stages of recovery showed considerable improvement in 'depression levels, anxiety, restful sleep, [increased] appetite, nutritional intake, energy and withdrawal symptoms'.[8]

ME (Myalgic Encephalomyelitis)

There is no known scientific research on the uses of Aloe *vera* with ME. There is, however, some anecdotal evidence which suggests an increase of energy in ME sufferers after using Aloe *vera*. Lady Elizabeth Anson said that it was Aloe *vera* which gave her a new lease of life after suffering from ME for years. She has set up a charity for ME sufferers which recommends the use of Aloe *vera*, alongside other natural treatments. Dr Anne Macintyre, herself an ME sufferer, reports that Aloe *vera* has achieved publicity as a cure for ME or CFS (Chronic Fatigue Syndrome) but that no trials have been carried out as yet. She suggests that Aloe's anti-fungal properties may be of relevance. ME can be linked to poor digestive processes where the body is deprived of nutrients and therefore fatigue and exhaustion sets in. As Aloe *vera* is effective in healing digestive problems, it follows that it will thereby increase the energy and vitality of the individual using it.

Multiple Sclerosis

Multiple Sclerosis is a disease of the nervous system which can manifest as forms of paralysis, walking difficulty, trembling eyeballs and hands and heavy depression with compulsive fits of weeping which alternate with laughing and extreme cheerfulness, to the point of hysteria. The causes of Multiple Sclerosis are unknown, although it can be triggered by stress. The type of person suscep- tible to Multiple Sclerosis is one who is prone to nervous diseases.

In Russia, work has been done by using injections of Aloe extract. The basis of this treatment is that Aloe stimulates the immune system defences and pro- motes vitality. This work has shown a successful outcome on patients suffering from Multiple Sclerosis with the use of Aloe *vera*.

Motor Neurone Disease

There is no known scientific work on the effect of Aloe *vera* in motor neurone disease. The authors know of one case, however, where the use of Aloe *vera* has been beneficial, although it has been used in conjunction with other remedies such as echinacea and St John's Wort.

Mark had been seriously ill with motor neurone disease for four years. After periods in hospital with life-threatening infections, he started taking Aloe *vera* with Neem. Aloe *vera* stopped the soreness of Mark's skin and eased the pain in his joints. The most remarkable effect is that Mark has not suffered with chest infections since he started taking Aloe *vera*. According to his wife, Natalie, 'He should not be here.' She also says that his 'complexion looks fantastic. Far better than all of ours!'

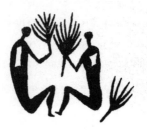

Aloe Vera in the Home

PART THREE

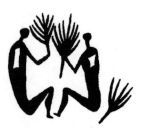

Safety Data

Caution

Do not use Aloe vera as a substitute for medical attention if symptoms are serious.
Before using Aloe vera plant or juice/gel etc., check contraindications – see below.

NOTE

Aloe *vera* juice and gel are here used interchangeably. Aloe *vera* gel is the juice with added thickening agent (such as carrageen). It is not more efficacious because it is thicker.

For People with Allergies

Aloe *vera* is recognized as being non-toxic in general, but it has occasionally been known to cause an allergic reaction in some individuals. Before using Aloe *vera* it is therefore advisable to check for possible allergies. Test by placing some juice or gel on the wrist or behind the ear. If a rash or stinging occurs within a few minutes, do not use Aloe *vera*. For most people, however, Aloe *vera* acts as an anti-allergenic when there has been an allergic reaction to other substances.

For Pregnant Women

Aloe *vera* should be used with caution, if at all, during pregnancy since it naturally stimulates the intestine which can produce a reflex response in the uterus. In the past, pregnant women were advised not to take Aloe *vera* internally as it could cause bowel spasms through its purgative effect. As it is the presence of aloin which causes this, only good-quality Aloe *vera* products – which use only the inner leaf gel, which have been properly stabilized and processed, and which should not contain aloin or only traces of aloin – should be used during pregnancy. In fact, in some cases Aloe *vera* juice has been used as a tonic with pregnant women with no side-effects. It can increase energy as well as digestive efficiency.

For Those with Cystitis and Gall-Bladder Problems

Those suffering from serious gall-bladder problems should not take Aloe *vera*. Nor should people suffering from cystitis or uterine haemorrhages use Aloe *vera*, as this can have an adverse effect.

For Those with Diabetes

People with diabetes should always consult their doctor before taking Aloe *vera* juice, as it may improve the ability of the pancreas to create more of its own insulin. Too much insulin is unsafe and therefore this should be monitored carefully by a doctor. In some cases people with diabetes who are taking Aloe *vera* juice have been able to reduce substantially the amount of insulin they require.

General Warning

The following is a list of ailments which have been known to respond favourably to the use of Aloe *vera*. As scientific research into Aloe *vera* is still in its infancy, only certain areas of its healing capacity have authoritative medical backing. Others have been traditional folk remedies in different cultures over the ages.

The authors take no responsibility for the efficacy of the suggested first-aid and home treatments with Aloe *vera*, except to state that these treatments are presented here for educational purposes and have been effective for others. There are a number of Russian folk remedies included here, never before available in English. The Aloe used in these Russian remedies is not specified as anything other than 'Aloe'. The authors' view is that this probably refers to Aloe *arborescens*, widely used in Russia. Aloe *vera* is also used in Russia as well as Aloe *saponaria*. The range of Russian folk remedies, however, shows a deep familiarity with the plant and the benefits it confers.

Dosage and Quality Control

ALOE VERA

There is a bewildering variety of Aloe *vera* products available on the market today. Unfortunately it is not easy to differentiate between a good-quality product and one that has been adulterated in some way. Although price can be a guide – the more expensive the Aloe *vera*, the better the product – this does not always apply. In the end, the key to judging Aloe *vera* is by results. If there is no improvement in your condition, change the Aloe product and try another.

For therapeutic purposes, the most efficacious Aloe *vera* is that derived from whole-leaf Aloe. Whole-leaf Aloe *vera* contains three to five times more of the active ingredients than the inner fillet of the leaf. Furthermore, concentrated Aloe *vera* which has not been pasteurized with high heat is infinitely preferable to Aloe that has been processed with heat. Aloe *vera* requires some degree of preservation because its carbohydrate and glycoprotein constituents spoil rapidly, and the most common ways of doing this are heat-processing or cold-pressing. Cold-pressing is a more expensive process than using heat treatment, and therefore cold-pressed Aloe costs more – but it is a price worth paying to get the full therapeutic results. There are some companies who process their product not just once, but twice with heat yet do not indicate this on the label. Heating prevents any mould formation but effectively destroys Aloe's mucopolysaccharides. If a product is heated, therefore, the Aloe constituents still present will continue to function to some degree, but be aware that its valuable immunostimulant action is lost with the loss of the mucopolysaccharides.

Instead of using heat, preservatives such as sodium benzoate (extracted from benzoin, a tree gum used by herbalists) and potassium sorbate (derived from the green berries of the mountain ash or rowan tree) are sometimes used.

There are Aloe *vera* products available which are of little therapeutic use. This is largely because of their high water content. Under present regulations, water does not have to be mentioned on the label and therefore an Aloe *vera* product may constitute mostly water with only a tiny percentage of Aloe *vera*, yet still call itself 100 per cent pure Aloe *vera*! At the extreme end of the spectrum, the consumer may be using little more than water. This both deceives and offers little therapeutic benefit to the consumer, especially in cases of serious illness where Aloe *vera* could be helpful.

For all these reasons, a concentrated Aloe *vera* which has not been high-heat pasteurized and uses the whole leaf is recommended.

The other misleading factor is the addition of calcium or magnesium to change the product's carbohydrate content. Maltodextrin, a kind of sugar made from corn starch, is also added to conceal the fact that the solids in Aloe *vera* have been diluted.

There is also the danger of oxidization, which occurs if Aloe leaves are cut and left lying around when they are harvested. Ideally processing should begin as soon as possible – that is, within 36 hours of the harvest, even when cold storage is used with the leaves.

Generally it is claimed that the International Aloe Science Council (IASC) seal of approval is sufficient to guarantee an Aloe *vera* product. The IASC (which is based in Dallas, Texas) has done a great deal of good work in bringing together scientific research on Aloe *vera* and establishing its credibility with government organizations. The IASC is not an independent body and developed out of interested Aloe *vera* companies wanting to regulate the industry. To get an IASC seal of approval, however, a product has to contain only 15 per cent Aloe *vera* and does not have to state that it contains water. The key to testing whether an Aloe *vera* product has a high healing capacity is to try to ascertain the number of mucopolysaccharides (MPS) present. These can fluctuate wildly but are sometimes included on the labelling. Independent laboratory reports point out that some products have as few as 1,200 MPS per litre while claiming to be 100 per cent Aloe, yet others contain as many as 18,000–21,000 MPS per litre.

It is always possible when buying an Aloe product to ask to see any independent laboratory testing showing the MPS count per litre. When buying cosmetic products, check the ingredients to see that Aloe is at the top or near the top of the list in terms of percentage volume in the product. If it is near the bottom and the cosmetic claims to be Aloe-based, do not buy it as it will contain too little Aloe to be of real benefit.

The authors know of two excellent products which do not carry the IASC seal of approval (suppliers are listed in the Useful Addresses chapter). Their reason for not seeking approval is that they do not consider the standards maintained by the IASC to be high enough. It would be far more helpful to the consumer if it were mandatory for each product to state the percentage of Aloe *vera* actually available in the product, the method of processing and the mucopolysaccharides count (in a broad range, allowing for harvest fluctuation). The highest therapeutic value is found in products containing between 10,000 and 20,000 MPS per litre.

For topical use, the best products to use are those made from whole-leaf Aloe *vera* juice. Many ointments are made from reconstituted powder and can contain as little as 10 per cent Aloe *vera*.

Recommended Dosage

We recommend using a whole-leaf Aloe *vera* concentrate. As a general guideline, though, follow the directions on the product you are using and watch your tolerance level. Too much Aloe *vera* can lead to diarrhoea. As it is a powerful detoxifying agent, too much Aloe taken too quickly can also lead to rashes as the liver starts detoxing.

The suggested doses are for those using a whole-leaf Aloe *vera* concentrate. If you are not using this type of product you will need far larger amounts for the plant to be fully beneficial.

Note that the taste of the plant can vary depending on the season in which it was harvested. After a long, dry period the Aloe will be darker in colour and have a much stronger taste.

- Maintenance dose: 2 oz (50 g or 50 ml) per day (1 oz/25 mg/25 ml taken twice daily).

- Therapeutic dose: 4 oz (100 g or 100 ml) per day (2 oz/50 mg/50 ml twice daily).
- In acute cases of illness: 8 oz (200 g/200 ml) per day.

This is of course a broad outline. We know of cases where bowel cancer cleared completely when the patient took 4 oz of Aloe *vera* daily. Even 2 oz taken daily can have remarkable results, but this is with a top-quality product.

Growing Your Own Aloe Vera Plant

Aloe *vera* is a plant that thrives in warm, dry countries. It cannot tolerate frost, so if you live in a northern climate it is imperative to grow your plant indoors with a minimum temperature of 55°F/13°C. If you grow it indoors, plant it in good-quality compost mixed with sand, with plenty of crocks or pebbles at the bottom of the pot to ensure good drainage. Eventually you will require a very large pot, at least 18 inches/45 cm in diameter, to allow the plant to grow to full size. It is not difficult to grow, as the plant is fairly hardy and not at all temperamental.

As the full medicinal value of the plant manifests at maturity – that is, at around three to four years old – it is best to start with a good-sized mature plant, which can be as tall as 4 feet/1.2 m in height. If you buy a younger plant, try to find out how old it is and wait until it is mature before harvesting. Note that the plant grows slowly and needs little water. The chief danger with growing your own Aloe *vera* is over-watering. Water the soil only when it starts feeling dry – once a week should be enough. Add 1 or 2 cups/200 or 400 ml of water and make sure that the plant has good drainage at all times. In really hot weather you can soak the pot for a while, but make sure you have good drainage so there is no danger of rotting the roots.

If you underwater, on the other hand, the plant will signal its distress with thin leaves which collapse into the middle. Without sufficient water the plant absorbs its own, resulting in thin leaves. Simply add water if this is the case!

Make sure the plant always has lots of light. Without sufficient light the leaves go flat instead of curving upwards. Although the plant likes sun, it can go brown in very strong direct sunlight, in which case it needs more water.

It is sensitive to fluoride in water which can lead to brown spots appearing on the leaves. Use spring or mineral water if you live in a water fluoride region.

If you grow the plant outdoors, note that it likes both some sun and a lot of wind. Wind actually strengthens the succulent leaves. Indoors it would be good to have it near a door where it can get some draught, or by an open window when the weather is warm.

The plant develops 'pups' or new shoots. Separate these from the mother plant once they are a few inches high otherwise they will draw nutrients from the mature plant. Transplant and water well and leave for three weeks so that they can develop more roots. Propagation is thus very easy.

For Home Use

When you harvest the plant for your own use, always take an outside leaf near the bottom of the plant first, as this will be the most mature and therefore have the greatest curative properties. The cut to the plant will seal itself. To ensure the most effective healing, use both the whole leaf and its gel. Slice the leaf in half and use the gel portion directly on wounds. Otherwise, extract the gel by scraping the pulp and juice out of a split open leaf into a container. Wash off any sap, as this will be bitter and act as a cathartic (a purgative or laxative). Blend the juice and gel, then refrigerate immediately. This can last for up to four weeks in the fridge. Do not freeze unstabilized gel as this will destroy its nutrients, nor cook with Aloe *vera* at a high temperature. If you do use it in your cooking, do so over a very low heat to minimize nutritional loss.

For an Aloe drink, slice the leaves into small pieces and place in spring water. Leave in the refrigerator for a day. Take out the leaves and drink. You can add your own organic cranberry juice or fruit juice to make the drink more tasty and interesting.

A–Z of Natural First Aid and Home Treatments

Abrasions

See **Cuts and Wounds**

Abscesses/Boils

See **Furuncle**

Acidity

See **Indigestion**

Acne

The skin should be cleansed well, with either Aloe *vera* soap or cleanser. Aloe *vera* ointment or gel should then be applied directly onto the skin. If you have a plant, use the juice from the leaf of the plant in the same way. This should be applied several times a day for at least a month. As Aloe *vera* acts as an astringent, initially there may be some dryness of the skin. It may be a matter of days (or weeks in more stubborn cases) before the skin responds, but usually there is a marked improvement, with old scars gradually disappearing.

For scarring, long-term usage is recommended, with a reduced dosage twice daily of topical application after the first month or two (this will vary from person to person according to the severity of the acne). If the skin is already dry, it might be necessary to use an Aloe *vera* moisturizing cream to counteract further dryness. Aloe *vera* can be used on sensitive skins, but it is always worth doing a test first. Its effect on the skin is to combat infection, stimulate tissue regeneration and not only heal without scarring but also reduce existing scar tissue.

Internal use of Aloe *vera* gel can speed up the healing process but this is optional.

Aching Joints and Muscles

Aloe *vera* ointment or massage cream is very effective rubbed directly onto aching joints and muscles. Relief is usually experienced rapidly and the ointment can be re-applied as often as required without any ill effects.

Ageing/Mature Skin

Aloe *vera* is called the Plant of Immortality for the youthful looks it imparts. Its use is recommended in contemporary books on rejuvenation with the exhortation, 'If aloe were discovered today, it just might be declared the wonder drug of the century.'[1] Here then are two remedies from different cultures for preserving a youthful complexion.

Tamil Nadu Folk Remedy for Preserving a Youthful Skin

Cut a leaf from an Aloe plant which is at least 30 years old. Once cut, allow the green slime to ooze out of the leaf for 12 hours. Do not use this green slime. Cut slices off the leaf and use the jelly (gel) from the leaf directly on the face and hands. If kept wrapped, the leaf will not dry out. You will experience an instant face lift! Use regularly.

Russian Folk Remedy for a Youthful Complexion

1 tablespoon sour cream

1 teaspoon egg yolk

1 teaspoon Aloe juice

Mix ingredients until you get a cream. Put this on your face (and neck) like a mask, in layers – one layer at a time, waiting until one layer of cream dries before adding another. A brush can be used for this. Keep the mask on your face for 20 minutes, lying on your back. Wash off with warm water and then rinse with cold water. This mask is good for any type of skin.

Skin Spots

Brown skin spots appear on the skin as we grow older, particularly on those areas which have been exposed to the sun, especially the hands. Aloe *vera* applied regularly either as juice from the fresh leaf or gel, twice a day over a period of several months, appears to be effective in reducing or removing these spots.

See also **Skin Care**

AIDS

See page 77

Allergies (of the Skin)

Aloe *vera* reduces pain and itching, accelerates healing and is therefore very effective for treating skin allergies.

Apply the juice or gel directly to areas of irritation at least 2–3 times a day or as required to control itching.

A fresh leaf from the plant can be used in the same way, applying the gel straight onto the affected areas or simply laying the leaf over them.

Daily doses of Aloe *vera* have been shown to enhance the body's natural capacity to deal with harmful substances. A recommended dose would be 1 tablespoon of juice or gel daily (either fresh from the plant or from an approved product).

NOTE

For most people Aloe *vera* acts as an anti-allergenic, reducing their allergic reactions. As it inhibits pain it reduces itching. It must be noted that about 1 per cent of the population is allergic to Aloe *vera*, so it is always worth testing yourself first: place some juice or gel on the wrist or behind the ear. If a rash or stinging occurs within a few minutes, do not use Aloe *vera*.

Alopecia (Baldness)

Certain kinds of baldness such as *alopecia areata* have been successfully treated with Aloe *vera* gel, applied 2 or 3 times daily to the affected areas. Treatment should be for at least 3 months to allow hair growth.

Hair loss due to infections of the scalp respond particularly favourably. The Mexican Indians applied the juice directly from the plant onto their hair and scalp at night and washed it out again in the morning. This not only guaranteed thick, lustrous hair, but also healed scalp abrasions and guarded against possible hair loss. Aloe *vera* juice can be used directly to heal scalp diseases.

Russian Folk Remedy for Hair Loss

Take Aloe juice, garlic, birch tree juice, honey and egg yolk (quantities are unspecified). Blend all the ingredients together. Rub this mixture well into the scalp and cover your head with a scarf. Leave in for at least 1 or 2 hours (more if you have time) before washing your hair as normal and then rinsing with the liquid extract of either stinging nettles or birch leaves.

Alternatively, mix 4 oz (100 ml) of Aloe juice with 18 fl oz (half a litre) of dry wine. Bottle and leave standing for 2 or 3 days, shaking the mixture occasionally. Rub this into your scalp daily.

Anaemia

Russian research has shown that ferrugineous Aloe syrup – 1 teaspoon 3 times daily for 12 days – increases the effectiveness of iron in the body to combat anaemia. The Aloe acts as a biogenic stimulator in conjunction with the iron.

Animal First Aid

The importance of pets to the health of their owners, particularly in urban societies, is now well documented. Owning animals can prolong life, reduce depression and even help lower blood pressure! Aloe *vera*, which brings such great benefit to humans, works equally well with all animals since its anti-viral, bactericidal, fungicidal, anti-inflammatory and wound-healing properties function in exactly the same way. The use of Aloe *vera* is spreading amongst American and British farmers, while Aloe *vera* products are commonplace amongst veterinary ranges in Australia and New Zealand.

It is not possible to cover briefly the wide applications of Aloe *vera*'s use with animals. In the US, Bill Coats and veterinarian Richard Holland have written a substantial book covering its veterinary uses,[2] and in Britain the outstanding equine vet Peter Green BVSc, Cert EO, MRCVS has used Aloe *vera* for the treatment of post-viral syndrome in horses. In addition, David Urch BSc, MA, Vet MB (Cantab), MRCVS has been advising on veterinary treatment using Aloe *vera*. Here we will deal with a few common complaints, chiefly affecting those animals who have enjoyed the closest and longest relationship with human beings: horses, dogs and cats.

Horses

Horses have always enjoyed a noble place in the history and culture of humanity. As a form of transport, warrior in battle, tiller of fields, companion to courtly knights, the horse has always been a potent symbol of energy and the life-force itself.

Nerves

Finely bred horses can be very highly strung. Aloe *vera* has been found effective in helping to soothe nervous horses. In California, trainer and breeder Imogene Peal gives any of her horses who are nervous and perhaps confined in their stall 4 oz (100 ml) of Aloe *vera* juice in their feed. This has proved successful in calming them down.[3]

Cuts, Bruises and Sore Legs

For bruises and sore legs, rub Aloe *vera* gel 4 times daily into the horse's legs or hocks until relief is obtained. If cuts are deep, saturate a dressing with Aloe *vera* gel and bind for 3 days. Change dressing after 3 days if required. This will speed up the wound-healing process.

Sprains, Strains and Swollen Joints

Soak liniment with Aloe *vera* juice. Bind onto affected area. Change bandage once daily. If it is difficult to bandage the area, rub Aloe *vera* gel into the affected area twice daily.

If you have an expensive racehorse (or a racing greyhound, for that matter), money is no object and the injury is detected immediately, freeze 4 oz (100 g) of Aloe *vera* gel in a paper cup. Crush this frozen gel and apply, wrapped in a towel, to the area. Bandage and leave the animal to rest. Apply 4 to 6 times daily while the inflammation is acute.

It is also beneficial to give horses Aloe *vera* gel internally in conjunction with topical use. Suggested dosage is 2 to 8 oz (50 to 200 g) daily, depending on the size of the horse and severity of the condition. Larger quantities are better broken down into smaller doses, for example 2 oz given 4 times daily.

Coughs and Sore Throats

Use 2 oz (50 ml) of Aloe *vera* juice several times a day to soothe the throat and combat infection. If the cough is chronic or there is a serious throat infection it is advisable to put the Aloe *vera* juice into a spray bottle and spray right into the back of the throat. This is also effective for horses suffering from the more serious type of cough known as folicular pharyngitis. If the horse has thick mucus coming out its nose, spray Aloe *vera* directly into its nostrils: 3 squirts into each nostril, at least 3 times a day.

Hoof Injuries

Always clean the hoof thoroughly. Apply Aloe *vera* gel and bandage. Change daily until the hoof develops its normal hardness (up to 10 days). The Aloe will accelerate any wound-healing, combat infection and also help new tissue to rebuild in the hoof. If there is swelling in the fetlock, use Aloe *vera* bandaged over the area to reduce swelling and inflammation.

Laminitis (Founder)

Laminitis is a common complaint, frequently caused by eating too much grass. The horse suffers from lameness and a low fever. Toxins are retained in the horse's digestive system which lead to a loss of appetite, creating weakness in the horse. In the US, veterinarian Dr Frederickson (who specializes in equine medicine) has found that Aloe *vera* juice can act as an appetite stimulant, not only for horses but also for cattle and other grazing animals. With seriously ill horses he uses massive doses of a quart (2 pints/1.21 litres) of more Aloe *vera* juice, tube-fed to the horse. Improvement will be rapid using this method – sometimes within three days.

Post-viral Fatigue Syndrome (Leucopaenia)

Vet Peter Green recounts treating 14 horses suffering from equine post-viral syndrome with Aloe *vera* gel. The white blood cells in horses suffering from leucopaenia can drop to almost fatal levels. He treated them over three to five weeks, with a success rate of 11 out of 14 horses making a full recovery and returning to eventing, jumping and racing. In these cases the affected horses showed increased white blood cell counts. Normally most of these horses would not have been expected to recover. Dr David Urch has had similarly successful results, treating more than 100 horses with Aloe *vera* and achieving an 80 per cent cure rate.

SUGGESTED DOSE

■ 8 oz (200 g) Aloe *vera* gel daily in food for 3—5 weeks.

Dogs and Cats

Besides horses, dogs and cats have been the longest-standing companions to humans. Dogs and cats share a number of common complaints which can be successfully treated with Aloe *vera*. The dosage will vary according to the size of the animal.

Arthritis

Dogs have been reported to have shown startling improvement when their arthritis is treated with Aloe *vera* gel; there is no reason to suppose that this treatment would not prove equally successful for cats.

SUGGESTED DOSE

- 1 oz (25 g) twice daily for cats, added into food.
- 2 oz (50 g) twice daily for dogs, also added to their food until relief is obtained.
- Continue on a maintenance dose of 1 oz (25 g) daily for cats and 2 oz (50 g) daily for dogs.

Aloe *vera* ointment can also be rubbed into the joints to ease inflammation and pain.

Digestive Problems

Both cats and dogs suffer from digestive problems such as irritable bowel syndrome and colitis, in much the same way as human beings. Change the diet to a bland rice and white meat diet, with no dairy products. Add Aloe *vera* gel either to the food or water.

SUGGESTED DOSE

- For cats: 1 oz (25 g) Aloe *vera* gel daily for 2 weeks.
- For dogs: 2 oz (50 g) Aloe *vera* gel daily for 2 weeks.

- After two weeks, reduce dosage. Give cats $1/2$ oz (12 g) daily and dogs 1 oz (25 g) daily.

Fleas

Fleas can be commonplace in dogs and cats, and carry a number of parasitic and infectious diseases which often cause skin problems. Flea collars are rarely effective unless filled with strong orthodox pesticides, which may kill the fleas on your dog or cat but unfortunately are so toxic that they can make the animal sick and damage its nervous system. This applies to flea soaps, ointments and sprays, which can cause an allergic reaction in your animals. Fortunately, fleas have an aversion to citrus-based products and also to Aloe *vera*, which is an effective insect repellent.

TREATMENT

Wash your pet with an Aloe *vera*/jojoba shampoo. Rub Aloe *vera* juice or gel all over the animal. Alternatively, use Aloe in a spray form. Wash the animal regularly with an Aloe-based shampoo.

In severe cases of infection and hair loss caused by flea infestation, be sure to rub Aloe *vera* juice or gel on twice daily. An alternative is to spray the Aloe *vera* juice directly onto the coat of the animal and rub well in. Continue for a period of 2 to 3 weeks. Simultaneously, oral doses (1 to 2 oz/25 to 50 g daily for dogs, $1/2$ to 1 oz/12 to 25 g daily for cats), added to food, helps skin-healing and alleviates stress.

It is often more difficult to spot fleas in cats because of their thick fur. Cats will also often eat the fleas, which can lead to complications like tapeworm, in which case you should take your cat to the vet.

Ringworm

Ringworm is not in fact a worm but is a fungus. Aloe *vera*, with its anti-fungicidal properties, is very effective in treating ringworm – Aloe *vera* clears the problem up twice as fast as antibiotics.

Ringworm in cats is infectious and can be transmitted to children and dogs. It is characterized by the appearance of concentric circles, with the outer rings being the most infectious. It is best if the cat is isolated during this infectious period.

TREATMENT

If the ringworm covers a small area, shave the area and treat the skin directly. Shampoo the area affected every other day with Aloe *vera*/jojoba shampoo. Be sure to shampoo inwards towards the centre of the ring, as the outer rings are the most virulent. Treat the newly shampooed area with generous applications of Aloe *vera* gel or Aloe *vera* juice, sprayed directly onto the infected area. Also be sure to treat the surrounding areas with Aloe *vera*, to prevent the fungus spreading.

In addition, add 1½ oz (37 g) Aloe *vera* gel to your cat's food.

If dogs suffer from ringworm, treat in the same way as cats but add 3 oz (75 g) of Aloe *vera* gel daily to your dog's food or water.

Continue until the condition clears up and hair growth is healthy. Once clear, continue adding Aloe *vera* gel as a maintenance dose to the cat or dog food, reducing to slightly over half the original dosage.

Mange

Dogs are far less prone to ringworm than cats, and far more prone to mange, which is caused by a mite. Dogs with mange can infect humans, causing scabies. Mange can lead to serious hair loss and cause stress to the dog.

TREATMENT

Wash or bathe the affected area with Aloe *vera*/jojoba shampoo. Treat the skin twice daily with Aloe *vera* gel until the lesions are healed. Continue bathing the dog twice weekly in Aloe *vera* shampoo as a continuing preventative and to stimulate healthy hair growth in the dog.

If a dog has become badly infected, add Aloe *vera* gel to its food or water – 4 oz (100 g) daily, spread over 2 doses, until the condition clears up and healthy hair growth is apparent. Once the condition is clear, continue on a maintenance dose of 2 oz (50 g) daily.

Seborrhea

Seborrhea is a scalp disease which is also found in humans and leads either to dry, flaking skin (dry seborrhea) or greasy skin (wet seborrhea). It affects any animal with hair covering its skin.

TREATMENT

Shampoo the affected area twice weekly with Aloe *vera*/jojoba shampoo. If the animal suffers all over with seborrhea it will be necessary to give it a full bath, otherwise only wash the particular affected area. Use Aloe *vera* gel twice daily on the skin and simultaneously give Aloe *vera* juice twice daily in the animal's food or water (2 oz/50 ml per day).

Hyper-sensitive, Hyperactive or Hysterical Dogs

Just as Aloe *vera* has been effective in calming the nerves of highly strung thoroughbred horses, so it calms down hyperactive or hysterical dogs.

TREATMENT

Take your dog off commercially prepared foods, which undoubtedly contain toxins, and put him or her on a well-balanced diet with vitamin supplements to flush out toxins. Keep the dog away from household toxins, cigarette smoke and all de-fleaing agents. Herbs which calm human beings, such as valerian or chamomile, are effective in calming animals (use these herbs in extract form). Additionally, 1 to 3 oz (75 g) daily of Aloe *vera* gel (depending on the size of the dog) added to the water helps to calm the animal and stabilize its nervous system.

Hairballs

Cats, due to their persistent grooming, are prone to hairballs gathering in their stomach and leading to coughs, vomiting or blockage of the intestines. Treatment with Aloe *vera* has proved effective, acting as a laxative and lubricant and helping the animal to expel the hairball naturally.

1 or 2 tablespoons of Aloe *vera* gel taken daily for 2 to 3 days should clear the system.

Cystitis and Bladder Infections

Aloe *vera* has been found effective in cystitis in cats, where it is far more common than in dogs.

TREATMENT

1 oz (25 g) twice daily for cats; 2 oz (50 g) twice daily for dogs. Halve the quantities once the condition is clear. If Aloe *vera* juice is in the animal's daily water, this will keep the bladder clear.

Ear Infections

Both dogs and cats suffering from ear infections can be treated by cleaning the ear and applying Aloe *vera* gel several times a day.

Arthritis

Aloe *vera* juice or gel, taken daily over a period of at least 2 months, appears to be very helpful for arthritis sufferers. Regular doses of 1 or 2 tablespoons of the juice or gel, taken 2 to 4 times a day, is recommended. Drink it with some fruit juice and follow with a glass of water. Once pain and swelling have subsided the dosage can be reduced to 1 tablespoon morning and evening.

Alternatively a drink can be made from the plant itself which is more economical. Cut off a leaf from the Aloe *vera* plant. Peel the skin away from the colourless pulp. Rinse the pulp well, cut into small pieces and steep in a jar of water. Keep the jar in the refrigerator. Add more water as necessary. Repeat as needed, using the recommended doses above.

Aloe *vera* gel or massage cream used topically on aching joints and limbs is very effective in conjunction with internal use. Overall results vary considerably depending on individual cases and can be as rapid as a couple of days. Certainly pain and any inflammation will be reduced, but it is important to stress that a period of regular usage over at least 2 to 3 months is recommended for long-term improvement.

Asthma
Russian Folk Remedy

Boil some fresh Aloe *vera* leaves in water and inhale the steam. You can either cover your head with a towel or place a brown paper bag over the steaming bowl, cut a hole in it and inhale.

An easier method is to use Aloe *vera* juice in an atomizer and breathe in the cool mist. Asthmatics frequently find it difficult to inhale steaming mist, so this is preferable and less messy. Russian research shows that atomizers containing Aloe *vera* show extremely positive results with asthmatics and pulmonary tuberculosis sufferers.

Athlete's Foot

Apply Aloe *vera* ointment or gel generously to affected areas and cover with a plaster. Re-apply frequently until the infection clears up.

A leaf from the plant, split open and spread over the infected area, then bound in place with a bandage, can achieve rapid improvement – even within 12 hours.

Bad Breath (Halitosis)

If the condition is linked to infected teeth or gums, then rub Aloe *vera* ointment/gel onto the teeth or gums at least twice daily, after brushing the teeth.

If bad breath arises through digestive disturbances, *see* **Indigestion**.

Bed-wetting

Aloe extract, injected daily, is used by doctors in the former Soviet Union to treat children suffering from bed-wetting. Associated symptoms such as low spirits, poor appetite and an irritable nervous system also improved during the course of treatment as the bed-wetting diminished or ceased entirely. The conclusion was that the irritation threshold of the bladder was raised.

Recommended treatment is the regular drinking of 1 tablespoon of Aloe *vera* juice or gel each day, mixed with fruit juice. Give for a period of 1 to 2 months and observe the child's response.

Blisters

For blisters caused by burns, Aloe *vera* gel sprayed onto the blister has been found effective. Re-apply before the skin dries. Continue to re-apply frequently until rehydration has been achieved.

For blisters caused by tight-fitting shoes, etc. apply Aloe *vera* gel or ointment directly, then cover with a plaster. Repeat until the blister heals.

Blocked Nose

Aloe *vera* juice can be used to decongest a blocked nose. Use 5 to 6 drops at a time. Do not blow your nose for 10 minutes after application. Repeat 2 to 3 times daily until relief is obtained.

Blood Pressure

Aloe *vera* juice, taken daily, can lower blood pressure within a few weeks. It can also lower cholesterol levels by 12–14 points. The recommended dosage is 2 to 3 tablespoons of juice taken twice a day.

Boils

See Furuncle

Bowel Problems

See Irritable Bowel Syndrome

Bronchitis/Laryngitis

Aloe *vera* gel, in an atomizer, has effectively treated pulmonary tuberculosis in Russia. Linked with its anti-inflammatory action and its anti-allergenic capacity are its soothing healing properties, thus making it effective in the treatment of bronchitis. Do consult a doctor, however, as this condition can be serious.

Russian Folk Remedy

Prepare this mixture for a compress: 1 part Aloe juice, 2 parts honey, 3 parts vodka.

Wet a piece of liniment thoroughly with the Aloe, honey and vodka mixture. Cover the damaged area with liniment – if it is the lungs, cover the chest; if laryngitis, cover the throat. After covering with liniment, put first a layer of cotton, then wax paper and finally wrap with a woollen scarf. Leave until the condition improves, changing the liniment several times daily.

Bruises

Apply Aloe *vera* gel or ointment directly onto the bruise several times daily. Its anti-inflammatory action will reduce swelling and marking rapidly.

A cut leaf can be used directly on the bruise and bound into place until pain and swelling are relieved.

Bunions

Apply Aloe *vera* juice or ointment directly onto the bunions at least twice daily.

Burns (and Scalds)

This has been one of the most thoroughly researched and documented uses for Aloe *vera*. If the burn is serious, a doctor should be consulted immediately.

There are four degrees of burns:

1 first degree, when the skin is not broken

2 second degree, when there are blisters and the skin is broken

3 third degree, when all the layers of the skin are destroyed

4 fourth degree, when the skin is charred.

Aloe *vera* can be used effectively in all four degrees of burns, but it must be stressed that medical help should be sought immediately for all but first degree burns. For more serious burns, Aloe *vera* treatment can be used in conjunction with medical advice.

For a household burn caused by hot fat, fire or boiling water, Aloe *vera* is excellent for immediate relief. Aloe *vera* ointment, gel or juice should be applied immediately. If you have an Aloe *vera* plant, slice off a leaf, cut it open and lay it on the burn. The gel should cover the burn area. Keep the juice in contact with the burn. After a while the leaf will seal itself up. At that point, scratch its surface to allow more juice to bleed out onto the burn. If the wound is kept wet for 48 hours, recovery should be excellent, with little or no pain or scarring. The Aloe will speed up the healing process and reduce the chance of any infection.

NOTE

If the burn is caused by acid, the affected area should be washed clean of the acid first before applying the Aloe *vera*. Otherwise application can be directly onto the burn.

Cancer

Naturally, cancer requires medical help. Some skin cancer sufferers, however, have found that using Aloe *vera* juice 2 to 4 times a day for several months has eliminated the cancer. In other cases, Aloe *vera* taken daily as a tonic will boost the immune system without any ill-effects.

For side-effects from radiation treatment, Aloe *vera* gel rubbed on to the affected area before and after treatment reduces pain and possible scarring. *See also* **Radiation Burns.**

Russian Folk Remedies

For General Physical Weakness

As cancer patients need plenty of vitamins and nutrients, the following treatments are recommended:

>4 oz/100 g Aloe juice
>
>20 oz/500 g ground walnuts
>
>12 oz/300 g honey

Mix all together and keep the mixture in a cool, dark place for 1 month.[4] After this time, take 1 tablespoon 3 times a day, 30 minutes before meals.

>2 glasses/400 ml/³/₄ pint Aloe juice
>
>2 glasses/400 ml/³/₄ pint beetroot juice
>
>2 glasses/400 ml/³/₄ pint carrot juice
>
>2 glasses/400 ml/³/₄ pint black radish juice
>
>2 glasses/400 ml/³/₄ pint klukva juice
>
>Klukva berries are bright red and similar to cranberries, but larger and with a more acidic juice. These berries grow in low bushes in marshy areas in the northern parts of European Russia and the Tundra

in Siberia. The juice can be purchased in most supermarkets, where it will appear under the name cranberry juice.

2 glasses/400 ml/³/₄ pint blackcurrant juice

2 glasses/400 ml/³/₄ pint birch juice (which can only be collected in very early spring by cutting the trunk)

2 glasses/400 ml/³/₄ pint St John's Wort (juice from the leaves only)

juice of 10 lemons

4 oz/200 ml spirit (such as vodka)

20 oz/500 g honey

Mix all ingredients together thoroughly. Put in a dark bottle in a dark, cold place for 3 weeks, shaking the mixture occasionally. Strain through muslin. Take 1 oz/30 g 3 times a day, 30 minutes before meals.

6 oz/150 ml Aloe juice

4 oz/100 ml juice from the leaves of May strawberries

10 oz/250 ml maple juice

10 oz/250 g honey

14 oz/350 ml red wine

Mix all ingredients together and store in a cool, dark place for 2 weeks. Take 1 oz/30 g 3 times daily, 30 minutes before meals.

40 oz/1 kg honey

1 glass/200 ml/^{1}/$_3$ pint Aloe juice

2 glasses 400 ml/^{3}/$_4$ pint birch juice

1 oz/25 g ground fresh birch buds

1 oz/25 g St John's Wort flowers

4 oz/100 ml vegetable oil

Melt the honey in a pot without boiling it. Add the Aloe juice and let the mixture simmer for 10 minutes on a low heat. In a separate container, simmer the birch buds and St John's Wort flowers in the birch juice for 10 minutes. Cover tightly with a lid and put in a warm place for 1 hour. Filter through muslin, squeezing through all the ingredients and liquid. Take the liquid and add to the honey and Aloe juice mixture. Stir thoroughly. Add the vegetable oil. Put mixture into dark glass bottles. Shake before using, and take 3 or 4 times daily, 30 minutes before meals.

The collection of birch buds and St John's Wort flowers (or leaves, as in the remedy on page 118) will involve going to the tree or plants themselves, although there are herbalists who carry St John's Wort leaves and flowers.

For Stomach Cancer

This is an extremely serious condition, but there is a remedy which has been used in Russia for well-developed stomach cancer when there is not much hope of an orthodox medical cure.

Take the leaves from an Aloe (not younger than 3 years old). Keep them in a cold (43–46°F/6–8°C), dark place for 10 to 12 days. After that, chop the leaves finely and squeeze the juice out. Put to one side.

Take 3 fresh leaves of pink geranium. Wash these in 3 tablespoons boiling water. Place in a heat-proof container, cover tightly and place in a boiling pan of water for 8 hours. Filter, then add this pink geranium liquid to a mixture made up of two teaspoons of the squeezed Aloe juice plus 18 oz/half a litre of cognac. Add 3 drops of iodine (5 per cent iodine).

Take 1 tablespoon twice daily, morning and evening before meals. In a few days there will be some pain, especially during the night. In a while the pains disappear and a stable improvement in the condition takes place. The pain does not return. This is the sign of the beginning of the healing process.

Candida

Aloe *vera* reduces infection and can be used directly in the vagina to obtain relief. Apply the gel several times daily to reduce itching. The juice can also be taken internally – 2 tablespoons twice daily.

Catarrh

Drink 2 tablespoons of Aloe *vera* juice twice daily until the catarrh clears up.

Chapped Skin

Apply Aloe *vera* ointment or gel directly to the affected area to soften and moisturize the skin. Continue to apply frequently until the condition improves.

Chicken Pox

Take 1 to 2 tablespoons Aloe *vera* juice or gel twice daily. Use fresh Aloe leaves
or Aloe *vera* ointment on the affected skin. Apply frequently.

NOTE

Dosage levels will vary according to the age of the child. Start with very small
amounts and increase the dosage until effective results show.

Suggested dosage would be half the adult dose for children up to 10 years of
age and three-quarters of the adult dose for children 10 to 14 years of age.
Children over 15 can take the adult doses suggested.

Please remember, no one can overdose on Aloe *vera*!

Colds

Take Aloe *vera* juice or gel, 2 to 4 tablespoons twice daily, to boost the immune
system. Inhaling the gel through a vaporizer is also effective in clearing the head.

Russian Folk Remedies

There are several Russian folk remedies for the common cold (and for tuberculosis – the remedies make no distinction between the two). Three are included
here:

8 oz/200 ml Aloe juice

40 oz/1 kg lime tree honey

4 oz/100 g birch tree buds

2 oz/50 g lime tree flowers

1 oz/30 g chamomile flowers

8 oz/200 ml olive oil

Before preparing the mixture, cut and wash the Aloe leaves with boiled water. Put the leaves into a cold, dark place for 10 days. Melt the honey and add the chopped Aloe leaves. Put together in a separate steamer above a pot of boiling water to warm. Separately, add the birch tree buds and lime tree flowers to 2 glasses of water. Boil for 1 or 2 minutes. Filter this solution. Put the solution into the already cooled honey-and-Aloe mixture and stir together. In another pan, add chamomile flowers to 1 glass of water and warm just up to boiling point (but don't boil). Add to the honey, Aloe, birch tree buds and lime tree flowers mixture. Stir well and put into 2 bottles, topping up each with 4 oz/100 ml olive oil. Store in a cool place.

Shake before using and take 1 tablespoon 3 times a day.

20 oz/1 litre pure spirit

4 Aloe stems

Place Aloe stems in the spirit and infuse for 4 days.

Take 40 drops 3 times daily.

1 bottle of wine

4 Aloe stems

Marinate the stems in the wine for 4 days.

Take 1 sherry glassful of this mixture 3 times a day.

See also **Asthma**

Cold Sores (Herpes Simplex)

Apply Aloe *vera* gel directly onto the cold sore several times daily.

Alternatively, place frozen Aloe juice on the surface of the cold sore. This remedy can also be used for warts.

Colitis

Colitis is a chronic inflammation of the digestive system which Aloe *vera* has been known to relieve. Take 2 to 3 tablespoons of Aloe *vera* juice or gel each day and monitor the results.

Conjunctivitis

Mix half Aloe *vera* juice with half water and use as eye drops. This has been used as a home remedy for hundreds of years, and is useful for general eye infections.

See also **Eye Infections/Inflammation**

Constipation

For centuries, Aloe *vera* has been used for its purgative qualities. A few table-spoons of juice or gel used daily keeps the bowels and intestines functioning effectively.

The aloin between the skin and pulp of the Aloe *vera* plant is the real purga-tive. If a stronger effect is needed, this is the part of the leaf to use. Peel the green Aloe *vera* leaves and place in a jar of water. Refrigerate. Drink a little of this twice weekly. For an even stronger cathartic use more green peelings, but proceed with some caution!

Russian Folk Remedy

Dry out the juice from a mixture of Aloes to make a brown-black powder, known as *sabur* in Russian, which smells unpleasant and leaves a bitter taste. It can be easily dissolved in 60 per cent spirit. Take 0.03 to 0.1 g (1 mg) before going to bed. Effects will be felt within 8 to 12 hours.

CONTRA-INDICATIONS

Don't take this if you are pregnant, menstruating, suffer from haemorrhoids or cystitis or have a bleeding intestine.

Corns

Apply Aloe *vera* juice or ointment directly onto the corns at least twice daily.

Coughs

Drink 2 tablespoons of Aloe *vera* juice twice daily until the catarrh clears up.

Cradle Cap

Mix Aloe *vera* juice with alcohol (brandy is recommended) and castor oil. Rub on hair and scalp. Leave for several hours or overnight. Wash out.

Mexican Indian Folk Remedy

Apply Aloe *vera* juice directly onto the scalp and hair. Leave overnight. Wash out in the morning.

Cuts and Wounds

First clean the skin thoroughly where it is broken. Rub Aloe *vera* juice from the plant onto the affected area; the ointment or gel will be just as effective. Repeat until the skin heals over.

If severe, cover with a bandage soaked in Aloe *vera* juice or ointment. This allows the easy removal of the bandage. The Aloe *vera* reduces swelling, alleviates pain and promotes rapid healing, with little or no scarring. Apply fresh gel regularly until the cut or wound is healed.

If you are using an Aloe *vera* plant, slice a leaf open and scrape out the pulp or gel. Spread this on the open wound and cover with a bandage or dressing. Re-apply as often as necessary.

Dandruff

Mix Aloe *vera* juice with alcohol (brandy is recommended) and castor oil. Rub on hair and scalp. Leave for several hours or overnight. Wash out.

Mexican Indian Folk Remedy

Apply Aloe *vera* juice directly onto the scalp and hair. Leave overnight. Wash out in the morning.

Denture Sores/Toothache

Rub Aloe *vera* gel under dentures and along the side of the gums for relief. Re-apply as often as necessary. Fresh juice from the plant can be used just as effectively.

Use Aloe *vera* juice/gel as a denture soak overnight to prevent infection. Dentures are frequently a source of candida.

If you have a hole in your tooth and can't get to your dentist immediately, put a small piece of Aloe leaf into the hole. This calms down the pain and inflammation.

Use Aloe *vera* as an antiseptic mouthwash by gargling with the gel or juice.

Dermatitis

See Eczema

Detoxification
Russian Folk Remedies

> 2 teaspoons fresh Aloe juice mixed in a glass/200 ml/$^1/_3$ pint of water

Drink daily.

> $^1/_2$ glass/100 g chopped Aloe leaves
>
> 1 glass/200 g sugar
>
> $^3/_4$ glass/150 g honey

Mix together and leave for 3 days in a dark place. Then add 1 glass red dry wine; again leave for 24 hours in a dark place.

Take 1 tablespoon 2 or 3 times a day before eating.

See also **Liver and Spleen**

Diarrhoea

Ironically, though Aloe *vera* works well for constipation it also helps with diarrhoea. In both cases the digestive system is not functioning effectively.

Drink 1 tablespoon of juice or gel several times a day until the diarrhoea stops. The anti-bacterial and anti-inflammatory action of Aloe *vera* is gentle on the digestive system and will restore it to working order.

Dry Skin

See **Skin Care**

Digestive Problems

See **Constipation, Diarrhoea, Indigestion**

Earache

If the cause is unknown, seek medical advice immediately. As a home remedy, make up ear drops using half Aloe *vera* juice, half water, mixed. Use a few drops in the ear. Relief can be immediate. If not, repeat several times daily until relief is obtained. Seek medical advice if pain continues.

Eczema

Aloe *vera* is a time-honoured treatment for eczema dating back to the ancient Egyptians.

Drink 2 tbsp of the juice or gel daily as well as applying the juice or gel externally to the affected areas until there is noticeable improvement.

Eye Infections/Inflammation

Dilute Aloe 50/50 with water, as 100 per cent Aloe *vera* juice would sting the eye. Bathe the eye using an eye bath twice daily. Repeat until inflammation ceases.

See also **Conjunctivitis**

Fever

Aloe *vera* can help to ease skin rashes or redness caused by excessive heat in conjunction with fever.

Apply Aloe *vera* generously to affected areas to control irritation. Repeat as required.

Furuncle (Boil)

Apply Aloe *vera* gel directly to the boil, cover with plaster. Repeat as required or until the condition disappears.

Alternatively, cut one thick leaf of Aloe. Wash it, cut it lengthwise and use it to cover the furuncle. Bandage and leave overnight.

Gastritis/Intestinal Problems
Russian Folk Remedies

If you have gastritis, drink Aloe juice for 1 or 2 months, 2 teaspoons twice daily 30 minutes before meals.

3 oz/80 ml juice from freshly cut Aloe leaves
Pure spirit (95 per cent)

Mix in the ratio of 80 per cent Aloe juice to 20 per cent pure spirit. This produces a light orange-coloured liquid which is very bitter and becomes dark when exposed to air.

Take 1 teaspoon–1 dessertspoon (depending on the severity of the condition) 2 or 3 times a day, 20–30 minutes before meals.

Take for 15–30 days. This can be used to treat gastric problems, colitis or problems of the gut.

6 leaves of Aloe, chopped fine and squeezed to produce 4 oz/100 ml
juice
4 oz/100 g honey

Mix together. Take 2 teaspoons twice daily, 30 minutes before meals.

Genital Herpes

Apply Aloe *vera* ointment or gel directly to the affected areas at least twice daily or until the condition clears.

Genito-Urinary Tract Infection

Women can use a douche and men wash with fresh Aloe *vera* juice (4 oz/100 ml) mixed with 5–10 drops Propolis tincture and 5–10 drops grapefruit seed extract – if Aloe *vera* is concentrated, then dilute with water.

Women can insert Aloe *vera* gel internally as well.

Gingivitis

Gargle with Aloe *vera* juice or gel and water, or apply the gel directly to the gums.

Gum Inflammation

Rub Aloe *vera* gel or juice onto affected areas.

Russian Folk Remedy

4 oz/100 g leaves of Aloe, chopped very fine

Place the chopped leaves into an enamel pot. Cover tightly with a lid and leave for 1 hour. Then warm slowly over a low heat until the mixture starts to boil. Remove from heat once it boils. Filter the mixture and put it in a glass container with a tight top. Keep in a dark, cool place. Use to wash and rinse gums and mouth.

Haemorrhoids (Piles)

For centuries haemorrhoids have been treated by Aloe *vera*, which brings relief to the extremely uncomfortable itching and pain. The condition can be treated both internally and externally; in severe cases both courses of treatment are recommended.

Traditionally a small piece of peeled Aloe *vera* pulp would be inserted in the rectum. It is still possible to do this, albeit somewhat difficult as the rectum can resist retaining the pulp.

It is far easier to use Aloe *vera* ointment, inserted gently into the rectum and massaged in. The other alternative is to use Aloe *vera* juice in a syringe for insertion into the rectum. Both the juice and ointment are useful together in extreme cases. Applications should be frequent: at least after every bowel movement, after bathing and before going to bed. Relief can be immediate, but treatment should be continued even after the symptoms are gone.

In conjunction with topical application it is helpful to take Aloe internally. The suggested dose is 1 tablespoon several times a day in fruit juice. This will improve the functioning of the digestive system. It will also prevent constipation, which is a frequent side-effect of piles.

Hair and Scalp Care

A lot of hair-care products now advertise Aloe *vera* as a constituent but it is difficult to know how much Aloe is present or whether the name Aloe *vera* is used as a fashionable or commercial gimmick. You can always add your own Aloe *vera* juice to a shampoo, or use it as a conditioner.

As a conditioner use it in the same fashion as the Mexican Indians: Apply the juice directly from the plant onto the hair and scalp at night with water. Leave it to dry out overnight and rinse it clean in the morning. This guarantees thick, lustrous hair and a healthy scalp.

Russian Folk Remedies

For hair that is dried out and bleached by the sun, heat (i.e. heated rollers) or chemical processes such as colouring or perms:

1 teaspoon Aloe juice

1 tablespoon honey

1 teaspoon castor oil

Mix together and rub into the scalp for 30–40 minutes before washing your hair. After washing hair, rinse with chamomile or stinging nettle solution. Then rinse again with clear water.

Repeat this treatment once or twice a week until your hair regains its elasticity.

1 tablespoon chopped Aloe leaves

18 oz/half a litre water

Boil the leaves in the water for 10 minutes. When the mixture cools, filter it. Take cotton wool and wet it with the liquid. Rub into the scalp 2 or 3 times a week. Do not wash your hair after rubbing the mixture on your head.

Fresh Aloe *vera* gel can be used to guard against inflammation after hair removal on the face, legs or bikini line.

See also **Alopecia, Dandruff**

Hangovers

Aloe *vera* is excellent for hangovers and associated headaches.

Rub Aloe *vera* gel on the temples and forehead to soothe and reduce pain. This helps to reduce the sense of 'fuzziness' and promotes clarity of thought.

Drinking Aloe *vera* gel (2 tablespoons 3 times a day for at least a couple of days) helps detoxify the system.

Drink plenty of water.

Headaches

Rub Aloe *vera* gel on the temples to alleviate pain and inflammation.

Heat Rash

Aloe *vera* can soothe heat-inflamed areas.

Rub the affected area with the fresh leaf of the plant, split open.

Apply Aloe *vera* gel repeatedly until the itchiness stops and inflammation ceases.

Hepatitis

With a fresh Aloe *vera* plant, use 3 oz of the gel mixed with 3 oz of water and 3 teaspoons of salt. Bring to the boil with 1 oz cane sugar. Take by the teaspoon, regularly (up to 4 tablespoons per day if the liver is badly afflicted).

Ayurvedic Remedy

Mix Aloe *vera* with turmeric and honey to create a tonic for liver disorders. Drink 1 to 2 tablespoons twice daily, depending on the severity of your condition.

See also **Liver and Spleen**

Hives

See **Heat Rash**

Hysterectomy

Take half a tablespoon of Aloe *vera* gel, twice daily, as required.

See also **Menopause**

Immune System

To boost the immune system, try this liqueur devised by Raspail, a 19th-century French scientist and medical man. One poetic admirer called it 'a dream from Ossian's paradise that found its way into Mahomet's heaven, the most subtle and exquisite gestatory perfume that I have ever known.'[5]

Raspail's Liqueur

36 oz/1 litre alcohol (60 per cent proof)

$^1/_2$ oz/15 g angelica root

pinch/2 g calamus

pinch/1 g myrrh

pinch/0.25 g cinnamon

pinch/0.25 g aloe

pinch/0.25 g clove

pinch/0.25 g vanilla

pinch/0.25 g nutmeg

pinch/0.25 g saffron

Mix together, then leave the mixture standing in the sun for a few days. Filter it. For each litre of the mixture, add 32 oz/800 g sugar. The liqueur is similar to Benedictine.

Impetigo

Apply Aloe *vera* gel directly to the affected area of the skin. Repeat twice daily or as required until the condition clears.

For skin infections use Aloe *vera* ointment or the split leaf of the Aloe on infected area. Improvement can be as rapid as within half a day.

Impotence

The Russians have had positive clinical results treating impotence using Aloe injected subcutaneously.

Russian Folk Remedies

Here are three Russian folk remedies using Aloe to restore potency or improve sexual potency.

> Equal parts of the juice of Aloe, fresh butter, goose fat, honey and powdered dried rosehips (ground finely in a coffee grinder)

Warm all ingredients together in a pot (be careful not to boil), stir thoroughly and then cover tightly with a lid. Keep it in a cool, dark place.

Take 1 tablespoon of this mixture with a glass of hot milk 3 times a day, 30 minutes before meals.

Geese have a very high sexual drive and are therefore very potent. Goose fat has been used in folk remedies over the centuries. In Wales it is rubbed on the chest against asthma!

6 oz/150 ml Aloe juice

10 oz/250 g honey

14 oz/350 ml natural red wine (in Russia the term 'natural' distinguishes wine made with grapes from adulterated wine)

4 oz/100 g powdered rosehips (very high in vitamin C)

1 oz/30 g powdered parsley seed (known for its aphrodisiac qualities since Roman times).

Mix all ingredients together in a bottle. Keep for 1 or 2 weeks in a dark place, shaking periodically.

Take 1 tablespoon 3 times a day, 30 minutes before meals.

4 oz/100 ml Aloe juice

20 oz/500 g ground walnuts

12 oz/300 g honey

2 oz/50 g powdered parsnip root

Mix all together. Keep in a dark, cool place. Take 1 tablespoon 3 times a day, 30 minutes before meals.

Indigestion

The juice or gel of the Aloe can be very helpful in regulating the digestive tract. It is known to be helpful for both dysentery and constipation.

Take 1 or 2 tablespoons of the juice or gel, with fruit juice, several times a day to keep the bowels regular.

Inflammation (of the Skin)

See **Swelling**

Influenza

See **Colds**

Insect Bites/Stings

It is important to treat insect bites or stings immediately, particularly if you are bitten by a bee, wasp or scorpion. Jellyfish stings can also be effectively treated with Aloe *vera*. Medical attention may be required depending on the degree of sensitivity to the bite or sting.

The most effective treatment is to use the fresh Aloe *vera* plant if you have one. Split open a leaf and immediately lay it over the bite or sting. This will draw the heat out and reduce the pain and any swelling. It also counteracts possible allergies. If you delay in treatment, the poisons will start functioning.

If you do not have a plant, use Aloe *vera* juice or ointment. In summer a spray of Aloe *vera* juice is useful against mosquito or midge bites.

Aloe *vera* also acts as an insect repellent if it is rubbed on the skin.

Irritable Bowel Syndrome

Take 1 or 2 tablespoons of Aloe *vera* gel or juice several times a day. Once relief is obtained, continue with a maintenance dose of 1 tablespoon daily, taken at night.

Itching

Aloe *vera* is very effective for both mild and intense itching or burning sensations, and acts as a natural painkiller.

Use Aloe *vera* ointment or gel generously on affected areas.

If you have a plant, cut the leaf and split it open. Apply the gel to the affected area, binding it in place. Alternatively, simply rub the leaf periodically on the itching, burning area for immediate relief.

NOTE

Check for possible allergic reaction – see page 101.

Joint Pain

See Aching Joints and Muscles

Laryngitis

See Bronchitis/Laryngitis

Leg Ulcers

See Ulcers

Liver and Spleen
Liver Detox

2 oz/50 g Aloe *vera* gel

5 drops Propolis tincture

2 drops grapefruit seed extract

Take this as a daily dose divided into two portions, once first thing in the morning and once last thing at night.

French Herbal Remedy

This remedy dates back to the 15th century. The quantities are not always specified in the original recipe:

Mix together $^2/_3$ g Aloe with the hot juice of a decoction of wild celery root, parsley, fennel, strawberry and sporage plus $^1/_3$ g mastic.

Drink 2 or 3 times a week.

Mastitis
Russian Folk Remedy

For treatment of advanced mastitis with boils on the nipples when breastfeeding:

Chop the leaves of Aloe and put on the damaged area (that is, the nipple), covered with a bandage.

Change the bandage as frequently as possible and add fresh chopped leaves as often as possible.

ME (Chronic Fatigue Syndrome)

Take 2 to 4 tablespoons Aloe *vera* juice or gel twice daily over a long period until there is a return of energy and sense of well-being.

Menopause

Indian Ayurvedic medicine considers that Aloe *vera* is excellent for treating the menopause or pre-menstrual tension.

Take half a tablespoon of Aloe *vera* gel, twice daily.

Russian Folk Remedy

For constipation during the menopause:

> 6 oz/150 g fresh Aloe leaves
>
> 12 oz/300 g warmed honey

Cut off the sharp tips of the leaves, then chop the leaves finely. Add the honey. Leave standing for 24 hours, stirring occasionally. Then warm the mixture and filter.

Take 5–10 g (about half an ounce) every morning, one hour before breakfast.

Menstruation

Dr Robert Svoboda, the first Western Ayurvedic doctor licensed to practise in India, considers Aloe *vera* 'one of the best tools we have to help regulate the monthly cycle'.[6] It tones the female organs and is called 'Kumari', a word from Ayurvedic medicine that refers to a young girl, virgin or maiden, to suggest both the healthy energy of a young woman and that Aloe provides the energy of youth.

Svoboda recommends starting with 1 tablespoon of Aloe *vera* gel per day, mixed with pomegranate juice or a sweet juice such as grape or apple, or cooled hibiscus or fennel tea. Take at the end of a period (try to use an Aloe *vera* produce which is not preserved with citric or ascorbic acid). If the Aloe *vera* agrees with you, increase to 4 tablespoons twice daily and continue as long as needed.

Another Ayurvedic remedy is Aloe *vera* gel fermented with honey and turmeric to be used as a tonic for anaemia, lack of menstrual flow and poor digestion. It can also be mixed with apple juice or water.

For a fresh source, use 3 oz/75 g of the gel from the plant mixed with 3 oz/75 ml of water and 3 teaspoons of salt. Bring to the boil with 1 oz/30 g of cane sugar. Take by the teaspoon.

Mouth Ulcers

Aloe *vera* juice and gel are very effective for treating mouth ulcers: apply frequently on affected areas. Also take Aloe *vera* juice internally until the ulcers disappear (1 to 2 tablespoons daily).

Muscle Cramps/Strains

See **Aching Muscles and Joints, Swelling**

Nappy Rash

Wash the affected area with warm water, then apply Aloe *vera* gel gently. Repeat at each nappy change.

Nasal Congestion

See Blocked Nose

Nipples (Cracked)

See Chapped Skin

PMT (Premenstrual Tension)

Take half a tablespoon of Aloe *vera* gel twice daily, as required.

> *See also* Menopause, Menstruation

Pain Relief

Treat the source of pain (the burn, cut or ache) topically with Aloe *vera* ointment or gel.

Peptic Ulcer

There have been favourable medical reports about the use of Aloe *vera* for peptic ulcer treatment.

Drink 2 to 4 tablespoons of gel or juice several times a day (at least 4 times a day, preferably half an hour before each meal and before going to bed). Take with milk, rather than fruit juice, to make the taste more palatable.

Instead of commercially-produced gel or juice, fresh Aloe pulp can be eaten directly. Peel off the skin, rinse the yellow sap and eat the pulp. It can also be liquidized and drunk. The taste should not be bitter if the sap is removed carefully. Take 2 to 4 tablespoons 4 times a day, as above.

Once symptoms disappear, continue on a maintenance dose of 1 to 2 tablespoons 4 times a day. Even advanced ulcers can be treated in this way.

Poison Ivy, Poison Oak

See **Allergies (of the Skin)**

Prickly Heat

See **Heat Rash**

Pruritus

This extreme form of itching can be treated successfully with Aloe *vera* cream. It reduces itching and burning completely in most cases.

Apply cream regularly until relief is obtained.

In the case of the plant leaf, split it open and place on the inflamed areas until itching ceases and the skin is soothed.

Psoriasis

Psoriasis is generally considered incurable. Aloe *vera*, however, has been used to treat this condition with some success and, if it does not cure the psoriasis, Aloe can at least keep it under control. Both internal and external treatments are recommended for maximum effectiveness.

Apply the juice or ointment to the affected area several times daily. As Aloe *vera* has an astringent action, lubricate the skin with a moisturizer to combat dryness.

Take Aloe *vera* juice (1 to 2 tablespoons) twice a day.

Radiation Burns
Russian Folk Remedies

Place Aloe leaves in a cold, dark place for 12 days at 42–46°F/ 6–8°C. Squeeze the juice from the leaves after this time. Take 7 parts juice, 11 parts castor oil, 0.1 part eucalyptus oil and 11 parts lanolin cream. This makes a distinctive-smelling cream.

Apply to the skin 2 or 3 times a day. Cover with clean cotton gauze.

1 part honey

5 parts Aloe juice

Mix together. This mixture can be used either on the skin to prevent radiation burns when undergoing radiation therapy or taken internally (when mixture is freshly made): 1 teaspoon 3 times daily before meals for 1 or 2 months.

Research shows that these freshly prepared treatments are good only for a limited period. Russian doctors working with the fresh Aloe cream, whether kept at room temperature or in the refrigerator, stated that after several days the cream started to deteriorate, losing its potency.

Rashes

See **Allergies (of the Skin), Fever, Heat Rash, Insect Bites, Itching, Nappy Rash, Stings**

Rheumatism

Numerous rheumatism sufferers have gained relief by using Aloe *vera* both internally and externally. There has not been extensive medical research in this field, however.

Aloe *vera* ointment or juice rubbed on the affected areas relieves inflammation. Aloe is also beneficial to the circulatory system.

Take 1 or 2 tablespoons of gel 2 to 4 times daily mixed with fruit juice. Patience is required with this treatment, as it may take at least a couple of months before you see tangible results.

See also **Arthritis**

Ringworm

Animals have been treated favourably for ringworm with Aloe *vera*. So far humans have not been known to use it for this treatment but it may well be effective.

Apply Aloe *vera* gel directly to the affected area.

Scalds

See **Burns**

Scalp Problems

See Hair and Scalp Care

Scar Removal

Aloe *vera* gel or juice applied twice daily over a number of months can reduce or completely remove minor scars. The older the scar, the more perseverance is needed. Try over a period of up to six months for results. Combine with vitamin E for maximum effectiveness.

Scrapes

If the scrape is painful, rather than rubbing on ointment – which may exacerbate the pain – try spraying on Aloe *vera* juice, or use a split leaf of fresh Aloe *vera* over the grazed skin. Reapply the juice or gel frequently (or use another Aloe leaf) over the next 24 hours. Once the pain has been relieved, it might be easier to continue with Aloe *vera* ointment until healing is complete.

Sciatica

See Aching Muscles and Joints

Seborrhea

See Alopecia, Hair and Scalp Care

Shingles (Herpes Zoster)

See Chickenpox

Sinusitis

See **Asthma**

Skin Care

Use of Aloe *vera* is widespread in the cosmetic industry because of its excellent results in treating skin complaints. You can treat your own skin directly by using Aloe *vera* cream as a foundation or as a night cream. The fresh Aloe *vera* leaf, sliced open and left on the skin for about half an hour, both cleanses and moisturizes the skin. It can also help heal any skin problems or infections.

Russian Folk Recipes for Home Cosmetics

To improve the complexion: 20 minutes before a meal eat 2 small pieces of green Aloe leaf (1 inch/2 cm each). The leaves have to be cut from the lower part of the plant. Peel the skin off. Chew the Aloe pieces slowly and carefully.

For vitiligo (depigmentation of skin) and thread-veins: Take fresh Aloe or preserved Aloe juice, 1 teaspoon 30 minutes before a meal, 2 or 3 times a day. This normalizes the metabolic function.

For Greasy Skin

1 oz/30 g Aloe leaves, chopped fine until they become like porridge
6 oz/150 ml water

Add the water to the chopped leaves. Leave for 1 hour. Filter and use liquid to cleanse your skin. This not only gets rid of greasy skin but acts as a tonic and freshens the skin.

Vitamin Skin Mask for All Types of Skin

$1/2$ teaspoon Aloe juice

1 teaspoon honey

1 egg yolk

1 teaspoon castor oil

$1/2$ teaspoon lemon or orange juice

1 teaspoon blackcurrant or redcurrant juice

Mix together, add blended oats to bind all ingredients together. Put the mask on already-cleansed skin for 15–20 minutes. Wash with warm water, then rinse with cold water.

This mask acts as a biostimulant for the skin. It tightens the pores as well as nourishing the skin.

To combat premature ageing of skin: 1 teaspoon Aloe juice 2 or 3 times a day before meals. Aloe juice acts as an agent to improve the blood supply of the pelvis, which helps to produce sex hormones, which in turn prevents the ageing process!

See also **Acne, Ageing/Mature Skin, Allergies (of the Skin), Chapped Skin, Eczema, Sunburn**

Sprains

See **Swellings**

Stings

See **Insect Bites/Stings**

Stretch Marks

Rub Aloe *vera* gel over affected areas once or twice a day. As with scars, persevere up to a period of six months.

Styes

See **Eye Infections**

Sunburn

Try to prevent sunburn by using an Aloe *vera*-based suntan lotion and by limiting your periods in the sun.

If you are burned by the sun, however, lie down and cover yourself with sliced Aloe *vera* leaves. You can also spray affected areas with Aloe *vera* juice as often as possible, making sure you keep the affected areas wet. This cools the heat in the tissues.

Aloe juice mixed with a moisturizer keeps the skin from drying out further: the inflamed tissues will cool down and the skin cells stimulated to heal themselves.

Aloe *vera* cream or gel can also be used directly on burnt areas.

Swellings

Aloe *vera* has been used as a natural anti-inflammatory for hundreds of years to treat inflamed wounds, injuries, etc.

For swelling due to infection: if you have an Aloe *vera* plant, slice open a leaf and lay the exposed gel on the affected area. Bind in place for up to 12 hours. As a natural poultice, this draws out any infection and allows the wound to heal.

Alternatively, rub Aloe juice, gel or ointment into the swelling until it dies down.

If swelling is due to athletic injury or a sprain, then Aloe *vera* can reduce the inflammation and any pain or discomfort. Cover the swelling with Aloe *vera* pulp and bind it in place. Alternatively, rub Aloe juice, gel or ointment into the swelling until it subsides.

Teething

Rub Aloe *vera* ointment or gel on the gums to ease pain as required.

Tennis Elbow

See **Swelling**

Throat (Sore)

As Aloe *vera* is a natural anti-inflammatory, use the juice to gargle with twice a day if you have a sore throat. Gargle just before going to bed to allow its action to work throughout the night. You can also swallow the Aloe juice (try mixing it with fruit juice); sip slowly.

Russian Folk Remedies

For Sore Throat (and Laryngitis or Inflammation of the Trachea)

Cut the lower leaves of the Aloe. Wash with water, chop and squeeze out the juice. Mix this juice with honey. Add honey in the proportion of 1 part honey to 5 parts Aloe juice.

Take 1 teaspoon 3 times daily, before meals.

For the Throat and Respiratory System

Before cutting the Aloe leaves, remember not to wash them for 3 weeks. Take 3 pints/1.5 kg Aloe juice, 2½ pints/1.25 kg honey collected in the month of May, and 7 pints/3.5 litres red wine. Put mixture in large dark glass jars. Keep for 5 days in the dark.

Take 1 teaspoon 3 times a day before meals.

NOTE   .

As this remedy makes a rather generous amount, if you require a lesser quantity use smaller proportions of the ingredients accordingly!

Thrush

See **Candida**

Tonic

Aloe *vera* can be taken daily as a general tonic. The recommended dosage is 1 to 2 tablespoons twice a day, or try 2 teaspoons of Aloe *vera* gel in a glass of water or fruit juice, 3 times a day.

Russian Folk Tonics

> Aloe leaves, washed, chopped finely and squeezed for their juice (to
> make half an ounce/15 ml)
> 10 oz/250 g honey
> 14 oz/350 ml red wine

Mix together, then leave in the dark at a temperature of 39–46°F/4–8°C for 4–5 days.

Take 1 tablespoon 3 times a day, 30 minutes before the meal.

> Use Aloe leaves from a plant which is 3–5 years old. First keep them
> in a dark place at 39–46°F/4–8°C for 12–17 days. Wash the Aloe
> leaves, chop them and add boiled water, in the proportion of 1 part
> Aloe leaves to 3 parts water. Leave for 1 to 1$\frac{1}{2}$ hours to infuse.
> Squeeze the leaves to get the juice (to make 4 oz/100 ml juice)
> 20 oz/500 g chopped walnuts
> 12 oz/300 g honey

Mix together the Aloe juice, walnuts and honey.

Take 1 tablespoon 3 times a day, 30 minutes before a meal.

Toothache

See **Denture Sores/Toothache**

Tuberculosis
Russian Folk Remedy

> 6 oz/150 g Aloe leaves
>
> 20 oz/500 g badger's fat (or you can use pork fat)
>
> 1 oz/25 g peeled garlic
>
> 2 oz/50 g birch tree buds
>
> 2 oz/50 g honey
>
> 4 oz/100 ml cognac
>
> 6–8 eggshells from the white eggs of a hen (these eggshells have to be dried and powdered)

Thoroughly mix all the ingredients. Place them in a jar and keep in a warm place for 5 to 6 days, stirring occasionally.

Take 1 tablespoon 30 minutes before a meal, once a day. If necessary and the condition is acute, take up to 3 tablespoons daily.

Ulcers (of the Skin)

Medical literature reports on the successful treatment of skin ulcers with Aloe *vera*. There may be an initial increase in pain due to the increased blood circulation in the affected area, but this does not last. Aloe *vera* gel speeds up wound-cleaning and regenerative cell production, so that the area of the ulcer diminishes fairly rapidly (within 1 to 2 weeks). Of course results will vary according to individual cases.

Use both Aloe *vera* gel and Aloe *vera* ointment on the ulcers, treating the affected area several times a day.

Urticaria
See **Heat Rash**

Varicose Veins
Medical advice should be sought with varicose veins. As yet there has been no systematic medical research on treating these with Aloe *vera*. There are reports, however, that as Aloe increases circulation and has an anti-inflammatory function, it has been helpful with varicose veins.

Rub Aloe *vera* juice or gel gently onto the legs twice daily.

Take the juice internally as well as using it topically. 1 to 2 tablespoons taken twice a day accelerates Aloe *vera*'s beneficial action.

Verruca(e)
See **Warts**

Warts/Verrucae
Apply Aloe *vera* gel directly to the wart (or verruca) 2 or 3 times a day for up to 3 months.

Alternatively, place frozen Aloe juice (or Aloe *vera* gel) on the surface of the wart or verruca twice daily and cover with a plaster. Continue until the condition clears up. This may take some time.

Worms
French Herbal Remedy

Based on a 15th-century recipe:

Mix Aloe gel with honey. Take 2 tablespoons twice a day.

Wounds

See Cuts and Wounds

X-ray Burns

See Burns

Yeast Infections

See Candida

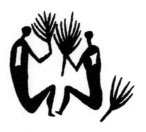

Further Information

PART FOUR

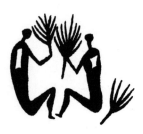

The Chemical Composition of Aloe Vera

Aloe *vera* clearly has many benefits:

- penetrates body tissue deeply, to seven layers deep
- naturally cleanses and anaesthetizes
- promotes growth of new cells and wound-healing
- encourages better tissue function and removes dead tissues
- acts as an antibiotic, fungicidal and virucidal
- acts as an anti-inflammatory
- stimulates and supports the immune system
- calms the nervous system
- cleans out the intestines and detoxifies the body
- has no side-effects, which may be connected to its synergistic action.

What qualities does Aloe *vera* possess which allow for such extensive healing to take place? Extraordinarily, in only approximately 1 per cent of the plant Aloe *vera* contains more than 75 nutritional compounds. As these compounds exist in minute amounts, contemporary medical research points to a possible 'synergistic' relationship between all the nutritional compounds of the plant, working together to create its so-called 'magical' healing abilities.

The charismatic reputation of Aloe *vera* in folklore is borne out by its chemical constituents. It is important to consider these components further to gain some understanding of Aloe *vera*'s powerful healing qualities. They can be roughly categorized as follows:

1 vitamins

2 enzymes

3 minerals

4 mono- and polysaccharides

5 lignin, saponins and anthraquinones

6 fatty acids

7 salicylic acid

8 amino acids

We shall now look at each of these categories in turn.

Vitamins

Vitamin A (beta-carotene)	Anti-anaemic, good for sight, skin and bones
Vitamin B$_1$ (thiamine)	Promotes tissue growth and increases energy
Vitamin B$_2$ (riboflavin)	Together with vitamin B$_6$, produces blood cells

Vitamin B$_3$ (niacin)	Regulates metabolism
Choline (a B vitamin found in lecithin)	Encourages healthy brain function and the metabolism of fats
Vitamin B$_6$ (pyridoxine)	Acts with vitamin B$_2$
Vitamin B$_{12}$	Traces of Vitamin B$_{12}$ have been found in Aloe *vera*. Aloe is one of the few plant sources of this vitamin, which is usually found in meat and dairy products. Lack of B$_{12}$ can cause anaemia and certain neuropathological disorders.
Vitamin C	Vitamin C (together with vitamin E) boosts the immune system and fights infection. Vitamins C, A and E are powerful antioxidants.
Vitamin E	Aids in healing
Folic acid (vitamin B complex)	Aids the formation of blood

Vitamins B$_3$, B$_5$, B$_6$ and B$_{12}$, in combination with certain minerals also contained in Aloe *vera* such as zinc, manganese and chromium, are positive for good brain functioning. All these vitamins are vital to general good health, and some are vital to the formation of certain enzymes such as vitamins B$_1$, B$_2$ and B$_3$.

Enzymes

Digestive enzymes are used throughout the body to allow chemical reactions to take place. In particular, the digestive enzymes help break down the proteins in our food into amino acids, which can then be converted back into body protein. The enzymes present in Aloe *vera* include the following:

Phosphatase	Aids in the production of energy in the body cells
Amylase	Helps digestion by breaking down fats and sugars
Bradykininase	Acts as an analgesic (reducing pain), as an anti-inflammatory (when used topically) and stimulates the immune system
Catalase	Prevents water accumulating in the body
Cellulase	Helps with the digestion of cellulose
Creatine phosphokinase	A muscular enzyme
Lipase	Aids digestive processes
Proteolytiase	Helps break down food
Fatty acids	Including caprylic acid, which is used as a fungicide (see below)

Minerals

More than 20 minerals are found in Aloe *vera*, including:

Calcium	For teeth and bone growth
Choline (a component of lecithin)	Needed for metabolizing
Chromium	Facilitates blood sugar levels, metabolizes glucose and aids circulation
Copper	Aids the formation of blood
Iron	Increases the body's resistance to infection and carries oxygen in red blood cells
Manganese	Maintains muscles and nervous system
Magnesium	Maintains muscles and nervous system. Prevents the formation of histamine from the amino acid, histadine. Histamine causes intense itching in allergic reactions. By preventing its formation, Aloe *vera* has an anti-pruritic and anti allergenic effect
Phosphorus	For teeth and bone growth
Potassium	Helps to regulate the fluid components in the muscles and blood
Selenium	Used in some very important anti-oxidant enzymes in the body
Sodium	Maintains (together with potassium) water

and other body fluids in balance. Transports
amino acids and glucose into the body cells.

Zinc   Boosts the immune system

Minerals are essential for the proper functioning of various enzyme systems.

Mono- and Polysaccharides

These are vital to the healing power of Aloe *vera*. The plant is rich in a class of long-chain sugars called mucopolysaccharides, known as MPS (these comprise both glucose and mannose – that is, the gluco-mannans.) These polysaccharides comprise:

- cellulose
- glucose
- mannose
- aldonentose
- uronic acid
- lipase
- alinase
- L. rhamnose
- acemannan

It is acemannan, in particular, in which Aloe *vera* is especially rich (it comprises approximately 90 per cent or more of the polysaccharides of fresh Aloe *vera* gel) and it works by boosting the immune system. It also stimulates white blood cells which destroy tumour cells and bacteria.

These sugars are derived from the mucilageous layer of the plant surrounding the inner gel. Taken orally, some of these sugars line the gut and help prevent 'leaky gut'. Unlike other sugars which are broken down before absorption, these polysaccharides are absorbed straight into the bloodstream in a chemical process known as *pinocytosis*. Here they act to enhance the immune system. Used externally, these sugars are the chief moisturizers of the Aloe *vera*.

Mucopolysaccharides (MPS) are normally found in each cell of our body and are manufactured in the first 10 years of our lives. Subsequently we look to outside sources for MPS, and Aloe *vera* provides a very rich source.

Lignin, Saponins and Anthraquinones

Lignin	Has a strongly penetrative effect with human skin
Saponins	Have cleansing, antiseptic and anti-microbial properties
Anthraquinones	Have analgesic and laxative properties and aid absorption in the digestive tract. Also have anti-microbial properties.

There are 12 anthraquinones found in the plant's sap. Two of the most important are:

1 Aloin

2 Emodin

Both are excellent painkillers as well as having anti-bacterial and anti-viral properties.

The other compounds are:

Barbaloin (Glycoside Barbaloin) and Isobarbaloin	Act as analgesics and have antibiotic properties
Anthranol, Anthracene and Aloetic acid	Act as antibiotics (without the toxicity)
Aloe emodin	Has bactericidal and laxative qualities
Ester of Cinnamic acid	May act as an analgesic and anaesthetic; also contributes to the breakdown of dead tissue
Chrysophanic acid	Has fungicidal properties for the skin
Ethereal oil (related to oil of ether)	Tranquillizing and analgesic
Resistannol	Believed to have bactericidal properties

What is most remarkable about the anthraquinones is that certain of them (emodin and chrysophanic acid), when isolated, show considerable levels of toxicity. Within the Aloe *vera* plant, however, they do not exhibit any toxicity. It appears that Aloe's water and nutrient content act as buffers against any toxic or allergic effects.

Fatty Acids

These are all unsaturated acids and are essential for healthy functioning. There are four of these plant sterols:

Cholesterol	Important anti-inflammatory agent
Campesterol	Important anti-inflammatory agent
B. Sisosterol	Important anti-inflammatory agent
Lupeol	Anti-inflammatory, antiseptic and analgesic

Salicylic Acid

Salicylic acid is made of a similar compound to aspirin and is a breakdown product from the Aloin found in the Aloe sap. It has anti-bacterial and anti-inflammatory properties.

Amino Acids

Amino acids affect brain function and are used to treat depression. They are also crucial to all bodily functions. There are eight amino acids found in the body, classified as 'essential' – that is, the body cannot manufacture them on its own. Seven of these eight amino acids are found in Aloe *vera*.

Furthermore there are 14 'secondary' amino acids, of which Aloe *vera* supplies 11.

Of the seven principal amino acids, five help in the assimilation of proteins; they restore blood cells; they prevent anaemia; they aid liver and digestive function, and muscle formation; they relieve insomnia, help cure depression and build up resistance to disease. The five are called:

- Isoleucine
- Leucine
- Lysine
- Methionine
- Phenylalanine.

This remarkable plant now has scientific and chemical explanations of its efficacy in a number of medical fields, knowledge which until recently was largely held as folklore. We know that it acts as an anti-inflammatory becauses of its fatty acids, cholesterol, campesterol and B-sisosterol; it controls (or eliminates) infections because of the natural antiseptic agents found in sulphur (known as a healing mineral for thousands of years), phenols, lupeol, salicylic acid, cinnamonic acid and urea nitrogen (another anti-microbial agent found in the sap). Pain is inhibited or completely relieved due to the presence of salicylic acid, bradykininase, magnesium and lupeol. While the enzymes provide penetrating power and the capacity to get rid of dead tissue, the amino acids provide a strong basis for healthy tissue to rebuild itself.

These are just some of Aloe *vera*'s qualities. Its most extraordinary property is its ability to respond appropriately to the needs of the person taking it. In other words, while taking it for arthritis it may simultaneously help a damaged liver. Or skin will noticeably improve while using Aloe *vera* to alleviate asthma.

Such a remarkably versatile plant can only have profound significance for our well-being as humans and also for the animals in our care.

References

ALOE VERA

Introduction

1. Dr Peter Atherton, *The Essential Aloe Vera* (Mill Enterprises, 1996): preface

The Aloe Family Tree

1. Christopher Brickell (ed), *Royal Horticultural Society Gardeners' Encyclopaedia of Plants and Flowers* (Dorling Kindersley, 1994): 432

2. Douglas Grindlay and T Reynolds, 'The Aloe Vera Phenomenon: a review of the properties and modern uses of the leaf parenchyma gel', *Journal of Ethnopharmacology* 16 (1986): 120

Myth, Legend and Folklore

1. Naveen Patnaik, *The Garden of Life* (Aquarian, 1993): 166

2. G A Stuart (revised from Dr F Porter Smith's work), *Chinese materia medical: Vegetable Kingdom* (Shanghai: American Presbyterian Mission Press, 1911): 30

3. Dora B Weiner, with a chapter by Simone Raspail, *Raspail:*

scientist and reformer (Columbia University Press, 1968)

4. Douglas Grindlay and T Reynolds, 'The Aloe Vera Phenomenon: a review of the properties and modern uses of the leaf parenchyma gel', *Journal of Ethnopharmacology* 16 (1986): 120

Traditional Uses

1. Prof J M Watt and Dr M G Breyer-Brandwijk, *The Medicinal and Poisonous Plants of Southern and Eastern Africa* (E & S Livingstone, 1932): 16

2. Watt and Breyer-Brandwijk, op cit: 15

3. G W Reynolds, *The Aloes of South Africa* (Johannesburg: The Trustees of the Aloes of South Africa Book Fund, 1950): 69

4. Al-Kindi, *The Medical Formulary or Agrabadhin of Al-Kindi* (translated with a study of its Materia Medica by Martin Levey; University of Wisconsin Press, 1966): 162

5. Frena Bloomfield, *Miracle Plants: Aloe Vera* (Century Publishing, 1985): 6

6. Col Sir R N Chopra, *Chopra's Indigenous Drugs of India* (Calcutta: U N Dhur & Sons, 1958): 61

7. Garcia da Orta, *Colloquies on the simples and drugs of India* (new edn; Lisbon 1895, imprint London: H Sotheran and Co, 1913)

The Age of Discovery

1. Cyril P Bryan (trans), *The Papyrus Ebers* (London: G. Bles, 1930)

2. John Goodyer (trans), *The Greek Herbal of Dioscorides* (Robert T Gunther [ed], Oxford University Press, 1934 & Hafner Publishing Co., 1968): 257

3. Goodyer/Gunther, op cit: 42

4. Pliny, *Natural History* (vol VII, with English translation in 10 volumes by W H S Jones; William Heinemann/Harvard University Press, 1949–1962): 399–401

5. Arthur J Brock (trans), *Greek medicine: being extracts illustrative of medical writers from Hippocrates to Galen* (J M Dent, 1929; reprinted 1977): 229

6. Frena Bloomfield, *Miracle Plants: Aloe Vera* (Century Publishing, 1985): 6

7. Frena Bloomfield, *Miracle Plants: Aloe Vera* (Century Publishing, 1985): 10

8. G W Reynolds, *The Aloes of South Africa* (Johannesburg: The Trustees of the Aloes of South Africa Book Fund, 1950): 62

9. Sir George Watt, *A Dictionary of the Economic Products of India* (vol 1 of six volumes; Delhi: Superintendent of Government Printing, 1889; reissued Delhi: Cosmo Publications, 1972): 186–9

20th-Century Advances

1. C E Collins, DDS, MD, and Creston Collins, 'Roentgen Dermatitis Treated with Fresh Whole Leaf of Aloe Vera', *The American Journal of Roentgenology and Radium Therapy* 33 (March 1935): 396–7

2. Creston Collins, 'Alvagel as a Therapeutic Agent in the Treatment of Radiation Burns', *The Radiological Review* 57.6 (June, 1935)

3. Thomas D Rowe, 'Effect of fresh Aloe vera jell in the treatment of third-degree Roentgen reactions on white rats', *Journal of the American Pharmaceutical Association* 29 (1940): 348–50

4. T D Rowe, B K Lovell and L M Parks, 'Further Observations on the use of Aloe *vera* Leaf in the Treatment of Third Degree X-Ray Reactions', *Journal of the American Pharmaceutical Association* 30 (1941): 266–9

5. Ibid.

6. R Y Gottshall, J C Jennings, C E Weller, C T Redman, E H Lucas and H M Sell, 'Antibacterial Substances in Seed Plants Active Against Tubercule Bacilli', *The American Review of Tuberculosis* 62 (1950)

7. Bill Coats and Richard E Holland, with Robert Ahola, *Creatures in Our Care* (Coats & Holland, 1985): 28

8. B K Rostoski, N Nordvinov and Max B Skousen, in *Aloe Vera – Quotations from Medical Journals* (UT: Aloe Vera Research Institute, no date)

9. Somova Levenson and Max B Skousen, in *Aloe Vera – Quotations from Medical Journals* (UT: Aloe Vera Research Institute, no date)

Aloe Vera as a Wound-healing Agent

1. Bill C Coats with Robert Ahola, *The Silent Healer – a Modern Study of Aloe Vera* (3rd edn; Bill Coats, [1979], 1996)

2. John P Heggers, Ronald P Pelley and Martin C Robson, 'Beneficial effects of Aloe in wound healing', *Phytotherapy Research* 7 (1993): 48–52

3. Dr Peter Atherton, *The Essential Aloe Vera* (Mill Enterprises, 1996): 16

4. Dr Lawrence G Plaskett, *The Health and Medical Use of Aloe Vera* (Aloe Vera Information Service, 1996): 24

5. Ibid.

6. Robert H Davis, Joseph J DiDonato, Glenn M Hartman and Richard C Haas, 'Anti-inflammatory and wound healing activity of a growth substance in Aloe vera', *Journal of the American Podiatric Medical Association* 84.2 (February 1994): 80

7. Robert H Davis, M Leitner, Joseph M Russo and Megan E Byrne, 'Wound healing – Oral and topical activities of Aloe vera', *Journal of American Podiatric Medical Association* 79.11 (November 1989): 559–62

8. Ibid.

9. Robert H Davis, Joseph J DiDonato, Richard W D Johnson and Christoper B Stewart, 'Aloe Vera, Hydrocortisone and sterol influence in wound tensile strength and anti-inflammation', *Journal of the American Podiatric Association* 84.12 (December 1994): 618

10. Robert H Davis, Mark G Leitner and Joseph M Russo, 'Aloe vera – a natural approach for treating wounds, edema and pain in diabetes', *Journal of the American Podiatric Medical Association* 78.2 (February 1988): 68

11. Ibid.

12. Ruth M Sims and E R Zimmermann, 'Effect of Aloe Vera on Herpes Simplex and Herpes virus (Strain Zoster)', Aloe Vera of America Archives, *Stabilized Aloe Vera* 1: 239–40

13. Bill C Coats with Robert Ahola, *The Silent Healer – a Modern Study of Aloe Vera* (3rd edn; Bill Coats, [1979], 1996)

14. Dr El Zawahry, Dr M Rasha and Dr M Helal, 'Use of Aloe in Treatment Leg Ulcers and Dermatoses', *International Journal of Dermatology* January/February 1973: 68–74

Skin and Hair Care

1. Albert Y Leun, 'Effective Ingredients of Aloe Vera', *Drugs and Cosmetics* June 1977: 34–5 and 154–5

2. Lawrence Meyerson, 'Open Letter', Aloe Vera of America Archives, *Stabilized Aloe Vera* II: 228 – from Bill C Coats with Robert

Ahola, *The Silent Healer – A Modern Study of Aloe Vera* (3rd edn; Bill Coats, [1979], 1996): chapter 7 ♪

3. Dr El Zawahry, Dr M Rasha and Dr M Helal, 'Use of Aloe in Treatment Leg Ulcers and Dermatoses', *International Journal of Dermatology* January/February 1973: 68–74

4. Tanweer A Syed, S Ashfaq Ahmad, Albert H Holt, Seyed Ali Ahmad, Seyed Hamzeh Ahmad and Mohammad Agzal, 'Management of psoriasis with Aloe vera extract in a hydrophilic cream: a placebo-controlled, double-blind study', *Tropical Medicine and International Health* 1.4 (August 1996): 508

Anti-inflammatory Properties

1. Robert H Davis, Joseph J DiDonato, Richard W D Johnson and Christoper B Stewart, 'Aloe Vera, Hydrocortisone and sterol influence in wound tensile strength and anti-inflammation', *Journal of the American Podiatric Association* 84.12 (December 1994): 614–21

2. Ibid.

3. O P Agarwal, 'Prevention of atheromatous heart disease', *Angiology* 36.8 (August 1985): 492

4. Neem oil is obtained from the seeds of the Neem tree which is widely grown in India. The oil has stimulative antiseptic and healing properties and has been used successfully for skin problems, ulcers and eczema. It is an excellent insecticide. Together with

Aloe *vera*, it has been effective in treating arthritis, diabetes, irritable bowel syndrome and stomach ailments including ulcers.

5. Jeffrey Bland, 'Effect of orally consumed Aloe vera juice on gastrointestinal function in normal humans', *Preventative Medicine* March/April 1985

6. Dr Peter Atherton, *The Essential Aloe Vera* (Mill Enterprises, 1996): 22

Aloe Vera and the Immune System

1. Dr Lawrence Plaskett, *Aloe Vera and The Immune System* (The Aloe Vera Information Service, 1996)

2. Ikuo Suzuki, Hiroko Saito, Shigeki Inoue, Shunsuke Migita and Taijo Takahashi, 'Purification and characteristics of two lectins from Aloe arborescens (Miller)', *Journal of Biochemistry* 85.1 (1979): 163–71

3. John C Pittman, MD, 'Immune Enhancing Effects of Aloe', *Health Consciousness* 13.1: 28 and 30

4. Lee Ritter, *Aloe Vera – A Mission Discovered* (Triputic, 1993): 14–15

5. Wolfgang Wirth, *Healing with Aloe* (Ennsthaler, 1995): 44

6. *The Times*, 1st May 1999

7. W D Winters, R Benavides and W J Clouse, 'Effects of Aloe extract on human normal and tumour, in vitro', *Economic Botany* 35.1 (1981): 89–95

8. Lee Ritter, *Aloe Vera – A Mission Discovered* (Triputic, 1993): 99

A – Z

1. Helene Silver, *Rejuvenate* (The Crossing Press, 1998): 101

2. Bill Coats and Richard E Holland, with Robert Ahola, *Creatures in Our Care* (Coats & Holland, 1985)

3. Ibid.

4. It appears that certain healing agents or biogenic stimulators (as yet unknown) are activated when the plant is kept in cold or darkness.

5. Dora B Weiner, with a chapter by Simone Raspail, *Raspail: scientist and reformer* (Columbia University Press, 1968): 135

6. Dr Robert E Svoboda, *Ayurveda for Women* (David & Charles, 1999): 147–8

Bibliography

ALOE VERA

Afzal, M, Ali, M, Hassan, R A H, Sweedan, N and Dhami, M S J, 'Identification of some Prostanoids in Aloe vera extracts', *Plant Medica* 57, 1991

Agarwal, O P, 'Prevention of atheromatous heart disease', *Angiology* 36.8 (August 1985): 485–92

Al-Kindi, *The Medical Formulary or Agrabadhin of Al-Kindi* (transl. with a study of its Materia Medica by Martin Levey; University of Wisconsin Press, 1966)

—, *Metaphysics* (State University of New York Press, 1974)

'Aloe Vera and Multiple Sclerosis' *The Valley Herald*, no date

'Aloe Vera. The Powerful healer' *Top Sante* October 1994: 45

Argument, Barbara, 'Cured by cactus juice!', *Evening Telegraph*, March 22, 1995

Atherton, Dr Peter, 'Aloe vera: magic or medicine?', *Nursing Standard* 12.41 (1996): 49–54

—, 'Aloe Vera: Myth or Medicine?', reprinted from *Positive Health* 20 (1997): 1–7

—, 'Aloe Vera Revisited', *British Journal of Phytotherapy* 4.4 (Winter 1997)

—, *The Essential Aloe Vera* (Mill Enterprises, 1996)

—, 'First Aid Plant', *Chemistry in Britain* May 1998

Barcroft, Alasdair, *Aloe Vera – Nature's Legendary Healer* (Souvenir Press, 1996)

Bissell, Frances, 'A–Z of Cooking', *The Times Weekend* April 10, 1999

Bland, Jeffrey, 'Effect of orally consumed Aloe vera juice on gastrointestinal function in normal humans', *Preventative Medicine* March/April, 1985

Blitz, Julian, Smith, James W and Gerard, Jack H, 'Aloe vera gel in peptic ulcer therapy: Preliminary report', *The Journal of the American Osteopathic Association* 62 (April 1963)

Bloomfield, Frena, *Miracle Plants: Aloe Vera* (Century Publishing, 1985)

Bovik, Ellis G, 'Aloe Vera: Panacea, or Old Wives Tale?', *Texas Dental Journal*, 1966

Brickell, Christopher (ed), *Royal Horticultural Society Gardeners' Encylopaedia of Plants and Flowers* (Dorling Kindersley, 1994)

The British Pharmaceutical Codex (Pharmaceutical Society, 1907)

British Pharmacopoeia (HMSO, 1907)

Brock, Arthur J (trans & annotated by), *Greek Medicine: being extracts illustrative of medical writers from Hippocrates to Galen* (J M Dent, 1929; repr 1977)

Brown, S., 'Aloe Vera. Could it be the Magical Ingredient in the Fountain of Youth?', *The Floral Magazine* August 1967: 35

Bryan, Cyril P (trans), *The Papyrus Ebers* (London: G. Bles, 1930)

Bryan, Mervyn, *Aloe Vera* (Healthwise Publishing, no date)

—, *An Introduction to Aloe Vera, the Complete Manual* (Aloe Vera Information and Advice Service UK, no date)

Budge, Dr E A Wallis (ed & trans), *Syrian Anatomy Pathology and Therapeutics or 'The Book of Medicines'* (vols. I & II; Humphrey Milford, 1913)

Chevallier, Andrew, *Encylopaedia of Medicinal Plants* (Dorling Kindersley, 1996)

Chopra, R N Col Sir, *Chopra's Indigenous Drugs of India* (Calcutta: U N Dhur & Sons, 1958)

Clifford, Terry, *Tibetan Buddhist Medicine and Psychiatry* (Samuel Weiser Inc, 1984)

Clumeck, Nathan MD and Herman, Philippe MD, 'Antiviral Drugs other than Zidovudine and Immunomodulating Therapies in Human Immunodeficiency Virus Infection', *The American Journal of Medicine* 85 (August 29 1988): 165–70

Coats, Bill C with Robert Ahola, *Aloe Vera, The Inside Story* (cassette tapes; Coats, 1997)

—, *The Silent Healer – a Modern Study of Aloe Vera* (1979, 3rd edn 1996)

Coats, Bill C and Holland, Richard with Robert Ahola, *Creatures in Our Care* (Coats & Holland, 1985)

Cole, Dr H N MD and Chen, Dr K K, MD 'Aloe Vera in Oriental Dermatology', *Archives of Dermatology and Syphilology* February 1943: 250

Collins, C E, DDS, MD and Collins, Creston, 'Roentgen Dermatitis Treated with Fresh Whole Leaf of Aloe Vera', *The American Journal of Roentgenology and Radium Therapy* 33 (March 1935)

Collins, Creston, 'Alvagel as a Therapeutic Agent in the Treatment of Radiation Burns', *The Radiological Review* 57.6 (June 1935)

Courtenay, Hazel, 'The cactus drink that may help cure millions', *Daily Mail* 14 April 1995

—, 'What's the Alternative' *Daily Mail* 26 September 1994

Crewe, J E, 'Aloes in the treatment of burns and scalds', *Minnesota Medicine* 22 (1939): 538–9

—, 'The External Use of Aloes', *Minnesota Medicine* 20 (1937): 670–73

Danhof, Ivan E, 'Aloe leaf handling and constituent variability', North Texas Medical Associates (no date)

Dash, Vaidya Bhagwan, *Materia Medica of Indo-Tibetan Medicine* (Sai-Satguru Publications, 1994)

Davis, Robert H, DiDonato, Joseph J, Johnson, Richard W D and Stewart, Christopher B, 'Aloe Vera, Hydrocortisone and sterol influence in wound tensile strength and anti-inflammation', *Journal of the American Podiatric Association* 84.12 (December 1994): 614–21

Davis, Robert H, DiDonato, Joseph J, Hartman, Glenn M and Haas, Richard C, 'Anti-inflammatory and wound healing activity of a growth substance in Aloe vera', *Journal of the American Podiatric Medical Association* 84.2 (February 1994): 77–81

Davis, Robert H, Leitner, Mark G and Russo, Joseph M, 'Aloe vera – a natural approach for treating wounds, edema and pain in diabetes', *Journal of the American Podiatric Medical Association* 78.2 (February 1988): 60–68

Davis, Robert H, Leitner, M, Russo, Joseph M and Byrne, Megan E, 'Wound healing – Oral and topical activities of Aloe vera', *Journal of the American Podiatric Medical Association* 79.11 (November 1989): 559–62

Davis, Robert H, Parker, William L and Murdoch, Douglas P, 'Aloe vera as a biologically active vehicle for hydrocortisone acetate', *Journal of the American Podiatric Medical Association* 81.1 (January 1991)

Davis, Robert H, Rosenthal, Kenneth Y, Cesario, Linda R and Rouw, Gregory A, 'Processed Aloe Vera administered topically inhibits inflammation', *Journal of the American Podiatric Association* 79.8 (August 1989)

Dirks Research, Ray (compilers), 'The Acemannan Report', *Health Consciousness* 13.1 (31 January 1992)

Di Sana Pianta, Edizioni Panini: 10, 150

Eliovson, Sima, *South African Flowers for the Garden* (Cape Town: Howard Timmins, 1955)

Espedal, Gunnar V, 'The Victorious Story of Viktor International', *Journal of Alternative & Complementary Medicine* March 1994

Fulton, J E Jr, 'The Stimulation of Postdermabrasion Wound Healing with Stabilized Aloe Vera Gel-Polyethylene Oxide Dressing', *Journal of Dermatological Surgical Oncology* 16.5 (1990): 460–7

Gerard, John, *The Herbal* (1633; ed. revd. and enlarged by Thomas Johnson, NY: Dover Publications, 1975)

Gjerstad, Gunnar and Riner, T D, 'Current Status of Aloe Vera as Cure-All', *American Journal of Pharmacy* 140 (1968): 62

Goodyer, John (trans), *The Greek Herbal of Dioscorides* ([50 AD, illustrated 512 AD by a Byzantine]; Robert T Gunther [ed], Oxford University Press, 1934 & Hafner Publishing Co., 1968)

Gottshall, R Y, Jennings, J C, Weller, C E, Redman, C T, Lucas, E H and Sell, H M, 'Substances in Seed Plants Active Against Tubercule Bacilli', *The American Review of Tuberculosis* 62 (1950)

Gottshall, R Y, Lucas, E H, Lickfeldt, A and Roberts, J M, 'The occurrence of antibacterial substances active against Mycobacterium tuberculosis in seed plants' *Journal of Clinical Investigation* 28.1049: 920–3

Green, Peter, 'Aloe vera extracts in equine clinical practice', *Veterinary Times* 26.9 (September 1996)

Green, Peter and Tong, Matthew, 'The Use of topical Aloe vera for the treatment of Skin Disorders in Horses', *Fellowes Farm Equine Clinic* March 1995

Griffith, F L and Thompson, H, *The Demotic Magical Papyrus of London and Leiden* (Clarendon Press, 1921)

Griggs, Barbara, 'Aloe, aloe ...', *Country Living* (March 1996): 122, 124

Grindlay, Douglas and Reynolds, T, 'The Aloe Vera Phenomenon: a review of the properties and modern uses of the leaf parenchyma gel', *Journal of Ethnopharmacology* 16 (1986): 117–51

Health Shopper, 'Aloe Vera – the rediscovered wonder plant?', *Health Shopper News* April/May 1995

Hedendal, Bruce Eric, *Whole Leaf Aloe Vera* (Beyond Nutrition Press, Offprint 17, no date)

Heggers, John P, Pelley, Ronald P and Robson, Martin C, 'Beneficial effects of Aloe in wound healing', *Phytotherapy Research* 7 (1993): 48–52

Heggers, John P, Kucukcelebi, Ahmet, Listengarten, Dimitri, Stabenau, Jill, Ko, Francis, Broemeling, Lyle D and Robson, Martin C, 'Beneficial effects of Aloe on wound healing in excisional wound model', Presented at 26th Annual Meeting of the American Burn Association, April 20–23, 1994

Heggers, John P, Kucukcelebi, Ahmet, Stabenau, Catherine J, Ko, Francis, Broemeling, Lyle D, Winters, Wendell, Bouthet, Catherine and Robson, Martin C, 'Wound healing potential of Aloe and other chemotherapeutic agents', Presented at the 6th International Congress on Traditional and Folk Medicine, December 1992, Kingsville, Texas

Henderson, Charles, 'Substance boosts therapeutic effects of AZT', *AIDS Weekly* August 5 1991: 2(2) – A and M University, Texas

Hennessee, Odus M/Cook, Bill R, *ALOE Myth-Magic Medicine* (Universal Graphics, 1989)

Hirata, T, Sakano, S and Suga, T, 'Biotransformation of Aloenin, a bitter glucoside constituent of Aloe arborescens, by rats', *Experientia* 37 (1981)

Hirata, Toshifumi and Suga, Takayuki, 'Biologically active constituents of leaves and roots of Aloe arborescens var. natalensis', Department of Chemistry, Faculty of Science, Hiroshima

University

—, 'Structure of Aloenin, a new biological active glucoside from Aloe arborescens var. natalensis', *Bulletin of the Chemical Society of Japan* 51.3 (1978): 842–9

Hodgkinson, Liz, 'Goodbye sickness, aloe vera', *Daily Mail* 29 November 1994

Hornsey-Pennell, Paul, with contributions from Dr Peter Atherton, *Aloe Vera The Natural Healer* (The Wordsmith Publishing Company Ltd, 1997)

Imanishi, Ken'ichi, 'Aloctin A, an active substance of Aloe arborescens (Miller) as an immunomodulator', Dept. Microbiology and Immunobiology, Tokyo Women's Medical College

International Aloe Science Council, Inc., *Official Definitions of Aloe*, IASC

James, Rebecca, 'Aloe Vera – Nature's Miracle Plant', *Alive* (no date given): 29–30

Kelvinson, Robert C, 'AIDS: a new frontier in research', Aloe Vera Information and Health Care Services, 1995

Krutch, Joseph Wood, *Herbal* (Phaidon, 1976)

Laidler, Percy Ward and Gelfand, Dr Michael, *South Africa: its medical history 1652–1898: a medical and social study* (Cape Town: C Struik, 1971)

Lawrence, Dr Derry, 'Treatment for Flash burns of the Conjunctiva', *New England Journal of Medicine* 311.6: 413

Leun, Albert Y, PhD, 'Effective Ingredients of Aloe Vera', *Drugs and Cosmetics* June 1977: 34–5 and 154–5

Livre des Simples Médicins, a 15th-century French herbal (introduction and adapted text by Carmelia Opsomer; English trans. by Enid Roberts and William T Stearn; commentaries by Opsomer and Stearn; Antwerp: De Schutter 1984)

Logan County News, 'Study treats Gum Disease with Aloe', June 1992

Loughran, Joni, *Natural Skin Care* (Frog Ltd, 1996)

Lushbaugh, C C and Hale, D B, 'Experimental acute radiodermatitis following Beta radiation', *Cancer* 6 (1953): 690–8

Macintyre, Dr Anne, *Chronic Fatigue Syndrome A Practical Guide* (Thorsons, 1998)

Marshall, Judith M, 'Aloe Vera Gel: What is the Evidence?', *The Pharmaceutical Journal* March 24, 1990: 360–2

Maughan, Rex G (presented by), 'The Miracle of Aloe', 20th World Congress of Natural Medicines in Madras, India January 25th 1991

Meek, Jennifer and Holford, Patrick, *Boost Your Immune System* (Piatkus, 1998)

Nadkarni, Dr K M, *India Materia Medica* (Popular Prakashan Private Ltd, 1954)

Natow, Allen J, 'Aloe Vera: Fiction or fact?', *Cosmetology* – Aloe Master International

Nutrition Update (Beyond Nutrition Press, Summer 1998)

Nutrition Update (Beyond Nutrition Press, Autumn 1998)

Obata, Masafumi, Ito, Shosuke, Hidehiko Beppu, Fujita, Keisuke and Nagatsu, Toshiharu, 'Mechanism of anti-inflammatory and anti-thermal burn action of Aloe arborescens (Mill.) var. natalensis Berger', Institute of Pharmacognosy and Comprehensive Medical Services, School of Medicine, Fujita Health University

O'Brien, Jim, 'Amazing Aloe', *Your Health* April 2, 1996

Patnaik, Naveen, *The Garden of Life* (Aquarian, 1993)

Pelley, Ronald P, MD, 'The Story of Aloe Polysaccharides', extract from *Inside Aloe*, official newsletter of The International Aloe Science Council Inc, January 1997

Pittman, John C, MD, 'Immune Enhancing Effects of Aloe', *Health Consciousness* 13.1: 28, 30

Plaskett, Dr Lawrence G, *Aloe Vera Information Service* (14 vols; Biomedical Information Services Ltd, 1996–7)

—, *The Health and Medical Use of Aloe Vera* (Aloe Vera Information Service, 1996)

Pliny, *Natural History* (vol vii, with English translation by W H S Jones; in 10 volumes; William Heinemann/Harvard University Press, 1949–62)

Ponce de Leon, Miguel, *Estudio de la zaabila o el aloe Maexicano* (Culiacan: Retes and Diaz, 1891)

Porter Smith, Dr F, *Contributions towards the Materia Medica and Natural History of China* (Shanghai: American Presbyterian Mission Press; London: Trubner and Co, 1871)

Priestley, Joan C, MD, 'AIDS and Aloe Vera extract', *Health Consciousness* 13.1: 40–1

Pulse, Terry L, MD, and Uhig, Elizabeth, R I E, 'A Significant Improvement in a Clinical pilot study utilizing Nutritional Supplements, Essential Fatty Acids and Stabilized Aloe vera Juice', *Journal of Advancement in Medicine* 3.4 (Winter 1990)

Reynolds, G W, *The Aloes of South Africa* (Johannesburg: The Trustees of the Aloes of South Africa Book Fund, 1950)

—, *The Aloes of Tropical Africa and Madagascar* (Mbabane, Swaziland: The Trustees of the Aloes of South Africa Book Fund, 1966)

Ritter, Lee, 'AIDS and Aloe Vera', *Health Consciousness* April 1991: 33

—, *Aloe Vera – A Mission Discovered* (Triputic, 1993)

Rowe, Thomas D, 'Effect of fresh Aloe vera jell in the treatment of third-degree Roentgen reactions on white rats', *Journal of the American Pharmaceutical Association* 29 (1940): 348–50

Rowe, T D, Lovell B K and Parks, L M, 'Further Observations on the use of Aloe vera Leaf in the Treatment of Third Degree X-Ray Reactions', *Journal of the American Pharmaceutical Association* 30 (1941): 266–9

Schauss, Alexander G, *Aloe Vera* (American Institute for Biosocial Research, 1990)

Semionova, N, *Aloe: the Natural Healer* (Moscow: Ripol Classic, 1998; orally translated from the Russian by Natasha Hull, 1999)

Sheets, Mark A, Unger, Beverley A, Giggleman, Gene F Jr, Tizzard, Ian R, 'Studies of the effect of acemannan on retrovirus infections: Clinical stabilization of felline leukaemia virus-infected cats', *Molecular Biotherapy* 3 (March, 1991): 41–5

Shida, Takao, Yagi, Akiri, Nishimura, Hiroshi and Nishioka, Itsuo, 'Effect of Aloe extract on peripheral phagocytosis in adult bronchial asthma', *Plant Medica* February 24, 1985

Silver, Helene, *Rejuvenate* (The Crossing Press, 1998)

Simon, David, *The Wisdom of Healing* (Rider, 1999)

Sims, Ruth M and Zimmermann, E R, 'Effect of Aloe Vera on Herpes Simplex and Herpes virus (Strain Zoster)', Aloe Vera of America Archives, *Stabilized Aloe Vera* 1: 239–40

Skokan, Stephen S and Davis, Robert H, 'Principles of wound healing and growth factor considera-
    tions', *Journal of American Podiatric Medical Association* 83.4 (April 1993)

Skousen, Max B, *The Ancient Egyptian Medicine Plant Aloe Vera Handbook* (Aloe Vera Research
    Institute, 1982)

Stow, G W and Bleek, D F, *Rock Paintings in South Africa* (Methuen and Co, 1930)

Strickland, Faith M, Pelley, Ronald P and Kripke, Margaret L, 'Prevention of Ultraviolet radiation-
    induced suppression of contact and delayed hypersensitivity by Aloe barbadensis gel extract'
    The Journal of Investigative Dermatology 102.2: February 1994

Stuart, G A (revd. from Dr F. Porter Smith's work), *Chinese materia medica: Vegetable Kingdom*
    (Shanghai: American Presbyterian Mission Press, 1911)

Sudworth, Richard, 'The Use of Aloe vera in Dentistry', reprinted from *Positive Health* 20
    (1997): 8

Suga, Takayuki and Hirata, Toshifumi, 'Biosynthesis of Aloenin in Aloe barbadensis var. Natalensis',
    Bulletin of the Chemical Society of Japan 51.3 (1978): 872–7

—, 'The efficacy of the Aloe plants chemical constituents and biological activities', *Cosmetics and
    Toiletries* 98 (June 1983): 105–8

Suga, Takayuki, Hirata, Toshifumi, Koyama, Fumihoro and Murakami, Eiko, 'The biosynthensis of
    Aloenin in Aloe arborescens Mill. var. natalensis (Berger)', *The Chemical Society of Japan.
    Chemistry Letters* 1974: 873–6

Suga, Takayuki, Hirata, Toshifumi and Odan, Michiyo, 'Aloenin, a new bitter glucoside from Aloe
    species', *Chemical Society of Japan. Chemistry Letters* (1972): 547–50

Suga, Takayuki, Hirata, Toshifumi and Tori, Kazuo, 'Structure of Aloenin, a bitter glucoside from
    Aloe species', *Chemical Society of Japan. Chemistry Letters* (1974): 715–18

Suzuki, Ikuo, Saito, Hiroko, Inoue, Shigeki, Migita, Shunsuke and Takahashi, Taijo, 'Purification and
    characteristics of two lectins from Aloe arborescens (Miller)', *Journal of Biochemistry* 85.1
    (1979): 163–71

Svoboda, Dr Robert E, *Ayurveda for Women* (David & Charles, 1999)

Syed, Tanweer A, Ahmad, S. Ashfaq, Holt, Albert H, Ahmad, Seyed Ali, Ahmad, Seyed Hamzeh and Agzal, Mohammad, 'Management of psoriasis with Aloe vera extract in a hydrophilic cream: a placebo-controlled, double-blind study', *Tropical Medicine and International Health* 1.4 (August 1996): 505–9

Taylor-Donald, Laurie, 'A runner's guide to discovering the secrets of the Aloe Vera plant', *Runners World* (1981)

Tchou, M T, 'Aloe vera (jelly leeks)', *Archives of Dermatology and Syphilology* 47, 1943

Tierra, Dr Michael, *Planetary Herbology* (Lotus Press, 1988)

Turner, William, *A New Herball* (1551; facsimile edition Cambridge University Press, 1989)

David Urch, *Your Questions Answered* (Forever Living Products, 1998)

—, 'Your Veterinary Questions Answered by our Advisory Board Member', *Forever 'IN-TOUCH'* September 1997

Visuthikosol, V, Chowchuen, B, Sukwanarat, Y, Sriurairatana, S and Boonpucknavig, V, 'Effect of Aloe Vera gel to Healing of Burn Wound, A Clinical and Histologic Study', *Journal of The Medical Association of Thailand* 78.8 (August 1995): 403–9

Waller, G R, Mangiafico, S and Ritchey, C R, 'A Chemical Investigation of Aloe Barbadensis Miller', Dept of Biochemistry, Oklahoma State University, Oklahoma, 1978

Watt, Sir George, *A Dictionary of the Economic Products of India* (vol 1 of 6; Delhi: Superintendent of Government Printing, 1889; repr Delhi: Cosmo Publications, 1972)

Watt, Sir James (ed.) with Clive Wood, 'Talking Health', Royal Society of Medicine Services, 1988

Watt, Prof J M and Breyer-Brandwijk, Dr M G, *The Medicinal and Poisonous Plants of Southern and Eastern Africa* (E and S Livingstone, 1932)

Weiner, Dora B, with a chapter by Simone Raspail, *Raspail: scientist and reformer* (Columbia University Press, 1968)

Williams, Xandria, *Liver Detox Plan* (Vermilion, 1998)

—, *Overcoming Candida* (Element, 1998)

Winters, Wendell D, 'Immunoreactive Lectins in leaf gel from Aloe barbadensis (Miller)'

Phytotherapy Research 7 (1995): S23–S25

Winters, W D, Benavides, R and Clouse, W J, 'Effects of Aloe extract on human normal and tumour, in vitro', *Economic Botany* 35.1 (1981): 89–95

Wirth, Wolfgang, *Healing with Aloe* (Ennsthaler, 1995)

Womble, Debra and Heldermen, J Harold, 'Enhancement of allo-responsiveness by human lympho-cytes by acemannan', *International Journal of Immunopharmacology* 10.8 (1988): 967–74

Wymant, Robert, 'Is this a cure for cancer?', *The Times Weekend* May 1st, 1999

Yagi, Akira, Harada, Nobuo, Chimamura, Koichiro and Nishioka, Itsuo, 'Bradykinin-degrading glyco-protein in Aloe arborescens var. natalensis', *Planta Medica* March 1986

Yagi, Akira, Harada, Nobuo, Yamada, Hidenor, Iwadare, Schuichi and Nishioka, Itsuo, 'Anti-bradykinin active material in Aloe saponaria', *Journal of Pharmaceutical Sciences* 71.10 (October 1982)

Yagi, Akira, Kanbara, Toshimitsu, Morinobu, Naoko, 'Inhibition of mushroom-tyrosinase by Aloe extract', *Planta Medica* 1987: 515–17

Yagi, Akira, Makino, Kenji and Nishioka, Itsuo, 'Studies on the constituents of Aloe saponaria (Haw.) II. The structures of phenol glucosides', *Chemical Pharmacology Bulletin* 25.7 (1977): 1771–6

Yagi, A, Makino, K, Nishiioki, I and Kuchino, Y, 'Aloe Mannan, polysaccharide, from Aloe arborescens var. natalensis', *Planta Medica* 31 (1977)

Yagi, Akira, Shida, Takao and Nishimura, Hiroshi, 'Effect of amino-acids in Aloe extract on phago-cytosis by peripheral neutrophil in adult bronchial asthma', *Japanese Journal of Allergology* 36.12 (1987): 1094–1101

Yagi, Akira, Shoyama and Nishioika, Itsuo, 'Formation of Tetrahydroanthracene glucosides by callus tissue of Aloe saponaria', *Phytochemistry* 22.6 (1983): 1483–4

Yeung, Dr Him-che, *Handbook of Chinese Herbs and Formulas* (vol i; Institute of Chinese Medicine, 1985)

The Yoga of Herbs: 100/101 (ch. Commonly Available Herbs) (printed sheet, no date given)

Zawahry, Dr El, Hegazy, Dr M Rasha, Helal, Dr M, 'Use of Aloe in Treatment Leg Ulcers and Dermatoses', *International Journal of Dermatology* January/February 1973: 68–74

Useful Addresses

ALOE VERA

UK

Aqua Oleum

Lower Wharf

Wallbridge

Stroud

Glos GL5 3JA

Tel: 01453 753555

Higher Nature

Burwash Common

East Sussex TN19 7LX

Enquiries and orders: (01435) 882880

Fax: (01435) 883720

Email: sales@higher-nature.co.uk

Nicholas Orosz

Aloe Vera Consultant

Aloe Vera Information and Products

17 Haldon Road

London SW18 1QD

Tel: 020 8874 7562

House of Mistry

15–17 South End Road

Hampstead Heath

London NW3

Tel: 020 7794 9848

Fax: 020 7431 5695

Email: mistry@dial.pipex.com

US

Aloe Life International

4822 Santa Monica Avenue

Suite 231

Santiago, CA CA 92107

Tel: [freephone from within the US

1-800-414-2563]/(619) 258 0145

Fax: (619) 258 1373

Website: www.aloelife.com

Lily of the Desert

1887 Geesling Road

Denton, TX 76208

Tel: (940) 566 9924

Fax: (940) 566 9915

Index